SURVIVING WORK-RELATED STRESS

Understand it   Overcome it

MELANIE KING

TRAFFORD

Cover photo by Adam Crowley from Getty Images.

Note for Librarians: a cataloguing record for this book that includes Dewey Decimal Classification and US Library of Congress numbers is available from the Library and Archives of Canada. The complete cataloguing record can be obtained from their online database at:
www.collectionscanada.ca/amicus/index-e.html
ISBN 1-4120-5465-6

TRAFFORD *Offices in Canada, USA, Ireland and UK*

This book was published *on-demand* in cooperation with Trafford Publishing. On-demand publishing is a unique process and service of making a book available for retail sale to the public taking advantage of on-demand manufacturing and Internet marketing. On-demand publishing includes promotions, retail sales, manufacturing, order fulfilment, accounting and collecting royalties on behalf of the author.

Book sales for North America and international:
Trafford Publishing, 6E–2333 Government St.,
Victoria, BC v8t 4p4 CANADA
phone 250 383 6864 (toll-free 1 888 232 4444)
fax 250 383 6804; email to orders@trafford.com

Book sales in Europe:
Trafford Publishing (uk) Ltd., Enterprise House, Wistaston Road Business Centre,
Wistaston Road, Crewe, Cheshire cw2 7rp UNITED KINGDOM
phone 01270 251 396 (local rate 0845 230 9601)
facsimile 01270 254 983; orders.uk@trafford.com

Order online at:
trafford.com/05-0363

10   9   8   7   6   5   4

About the author

After graduating with a degree in International Relations from Sussex University, Melanie King worked for two years in Thailand, first with hill tribe refugees temporarily housed in camps, then as a journalist on a national newspaper. She has worked and travelled extensively around the globe with jobs that have included helping victims of torture, writing CVs for Bosnian refuges, editing publications at the Royal Institute of International Affairs in London, and working in Brussels as assistant to the Director of the Institute for South and South-east Asian Affairs. In 1991, King trained as a careers adviser and spent 12 years advising school, college and university students in various settings. Based in Oxfordshire, she now works as a freelance careers adviser and writer.

For Bunny

Contents

Author's Note

This book offers general advice and should not be relied on as a substitute for proper medical or legal consultation. The author and publisher cannot accept responsibility for illness or loss of income arising from the failure to seek medical advice from a doctor or legal advice from a qualified professional.

All of the case studies in this book are based on real people, but their names and places of work have been changed to protect their identities.

Acknowledgments

I would like to thank my husband Ross, not only for his keen editorial eye but also for all his untiring support for the project, without which this book would not have materialised. I would also like to thank my dear friend Susan Adams for patiently reading through chapter after chapter, and for correcting some of my stranger sentence constructions. Her viewpoint from that of an employer has also been invaluable.

Thank you to Andrew Green D.C, from the Woodstock Chiropractic Clinic in Oxfordshire, who read through the section on chiropractics. Thank you also to Professor Jing Hua Chen, MD, L.M. BAcC, H.M RCHM, consultant to the Hale Clinic and the Integrated Medical Centre in London, who as a friend and outstanding acupuncturist offered suggestions to improve the section on acupuncture and treating stress.

Thank you to Duncan Midwinter for designing the cover and illustrations and to Dr. Barrington-Ward, Niamh Hyland, Toshio Nomura, Tim Field and Nick Williams, founder of Heat at Work London, co-founder of Dreambuilders Community and a trustee Director of Alternatives, for their kindness.

Thank you also Bunny, Destine, Steve, Ben, Andrew and Anne for believing in me.

Finally, but not least, thank you to all those who told me their stories, inspiring the creation of this book. I hope you will be an inspiration to others going through work-related stress, as you have been to me.

Is this book for you?

- Each day you come home from work exhausted and depressed.

- You feel unable to cope with your mounting work load.

- You have lost all enthusiasm and motivation for your job.

- Your self-confidence is waning.

- You feel ill much of the time.

- Your work colleagues are often off sick, and there is a rapid staff turn-over at your workplace.

- Those close to you say your personality has changed.

PART ONE

Unfulfilling vocations: The background to work-related stress and its effects

You are not here merely to make a living. You are here in order to enable the world to live more amply, with greater vision, with finer spirit of hope and achievement. You are here to enrich the world, and you impoverish yourself if you forget the errand.

Woodrow Wilson (1856-1924)

1 HOW BIG IS THE PROBLEM?

Each morning I would wake up full of dread. Dressing myself was a huge chore, as was preparing and eating breakfast. My hand would start to shake as I unlocked the car for the short journey to work. As I turned the office door handle, my heart beat so fast I thought I was having a heart attack.

Sally, 35.

If, like Sally, you are suffering from work-related stress, then you are not alone. According to a report released in 2002 by Amicus, the UK's largest private sector union, Britain's work places are becoming more stressful. Of the two thousand union health and safety representatives interviewed, half believed that stress was a much greater problem than five years previously, and that there were significant increases in the last twelve months.[1] A Health and Safety Committee report found that between 2001 and 2002, 32.9 million working days had been lost due to work-related illnesses.[2] Official government figures show that over a million people are claiming incapacity benefits due to stress, and that there are more than 200,000 new claimants each year. And the Doctor Patient Partnership (DPP) is so concerned about the escalation of work-related stress that in 2003 it launched a campaign to help people recognise and manage their stress.[3]

This epidemic of work-related stress is not just a problem for the individuals concerned. Such high volumes of stress have dramatic consequences for the country's economy as well. According to researchers at the University of Nottingham, the experience of work-related stress 'is a threat to the health of working people and to the healthiness of their work organisations.[4] The BBC reported in June 2001 that each day 270,000 people take time off work due to stress-related illnesses and that absenteeism cost the UK 10.2 billion pounds in 2000[5] – a sum greater than the Gross National Product of Kenya.

So what is going on in the 21st century? In an era of workers' rights, compensation culture, resurgent unions, and notions of work-life balance, are workers becoming too soft and their expectations unrealistically high? Are they the prey of pharmaceutical companies and the dupes of stress-management gurus? Or is the British workplace becoming dangerously ill, imperilling both the physical and economic health of the nation?

How much stress is good for you?

I used to think that someone who was off on long-term sick leave with 'stress' was scamming it. We all get stressed – stress is part of modern living. And then one morning I could not get out of bed. Pins and needles shot up my arms and legs and I literally went numb all over. It was the most frightening experience of my life.

Christine, 29.

What do we mean when we talk about work-related stress? The Health and Safety Executive (HSE) defines it as follows: 'Stress is the adverse reaction people have to excessive pressure or other types of demand placed on them. It can be caused by things at work or by things outside work, or both. Work-related stress arises from, or is made worse by, work.'[6]

Dr Hans Selye, the Czech-born father of stress research who died in 1982, defines stress as a wide range of strong external stimuli, both physiological and psychological, which in turn can cause a physiological response that he called the 'General Adaptation Syndrome'. The General Adaptation Syndrome has three distinct stages:

- Alarm reaction – the body detects the external stimulus
- Adaptation – the body engages defensive countermeasures against the stressor
- Exhaustion – the body begins to run out of defences

Selye differentiated between "distress" (negative stress) and "eustress" (positive stress). He claimed a little bit of "eustress" provides the stimulation that can inspire us to prepare in advance for, say, a difficult situation such as a job interview or an exam. On the other hand, it is the "distress" (negative stress) that should either be avoided or reduced. Selye argued that all sorts of things, whether little or large, can cause stress, and that positive experiences, such as getting married or promotion at work, can also trigger stress.

It is from Selye, therefore, that we derive the popular, but often misunderstood, belief that a little bit of stress is good for us, enabling us to work more efficiently. For instance, how many times have you heard a colleague say, 'I work much better if I leave everything to the last minute', or 'When I was at university I would stay up all night to get my essays in on time'? People who make such comments have developed a system of using "eustress" – playing brinkmanship with deadlines, for example – to motivate themselves to get the job done. The saying that a little bit of stress is good for you means that a moderate amount of the 'right kind of stress' can motivate us to take action. However, too much of the wrong kind of stress can seriously damage the health. And indeed, psychologists have found that even very low levels of stress can decrease performance in many people.

'Fight or flight'

The physical and mental effects of stress should never be underestimated. Stress causes a biological response that was genetically programmed into us thousands of years ago, to protect us when physical survival was dangerous. Our bodies would go into 'fight or flight' mode when danger threatened, such as a sabre-toothed tiger lurking outside the cave. In the 21st century the mechanics of the stress function are still in place and can be set off, often unwittingly. If you find yourself walking down a dark alley late at night and discover you are being followed by a group of aggressive youths, you will probably find that your heart starts pounding extra fast. The accompanying adrenaline rush in most cases will prepare you to run – i.e., take flight. According to researchers at the Harvard Medical School, the following physiological changes will occur as the sympathetic nervous system kicks in:

- Your heart rate, blood pressure and respiration rise to ensure an adequate oxygen level.
- Blood flow increases to the muscles and brain – where it is most needed – while blood flow decreases to the stomach and other organs that are less important in the moment of crisis.
- Sweating and muscle tension increase to help adjust body temperature and prepare for movement.
- Blood glucose increases to boost energy resources.

These physiological changes take place when your brain senses a threat, be it muggers, sabre-tooth tigers, or simply the thought of confronting a bullying co-worker. Signals are sent via your nervous system throughout your body, communicating that you are now ready to take physical action against the potential threat. This automatic mechanism may be useful if we need to run from pre-historic beasts or gangs of hooligans, but what about when it becomes our response to a job?

Stress in small doses does not, in most people, necessarily lead to ill health. The problem arises when it occurs over prolonged periods. People vary in the amount of stress they can take before it affects their physical and mental well being, but each of us has a responsibility to understand what levels we can safely afford. This might vary at the different stages of our lives, so it is extremely important to know our limits. It is also important to remember that suffering from stress is not a deficiency in character. Stress is not a weakness, as indicated by the fact that the very mechanism of the stress function – the fight or flight reaction – is part of our make-up as human beings, and is what has helped us to survive through the millennia. History is filled with famous high achievers who have succumbed, at one time or another, to ailments related to stress – the only difference being that the condition was not recognised. The first Duke of Marlborough, John Churchill, one of the greatest military commanders in history, suffered appalling headaches throughout his adult life, undoubtedly related to stress. Despite his sensational success on the battlefield – he never lost a battle – Marlborough wrote in 1711 that 'the dayly vexatons I meet with dose not only break my sperit but also my constitution.'[7] Likewise, Benjamin Disraeli, Queen Victoria's flamboyant and capable Prime Minister, also suffered throughout his life from stress-related illnesses such as depression, nervous exhaustion and violent headaches.[8] However, when Dr Selye, the pioneer of stress research, was asked to present papers on the subject in France and Germany in the 1930s, neither country had a word for it. In both instances, they coined words – 'le stress' and 'der stress' – to promote his work. You could say that the experience of stress was only acknowledged in the 1930s!

The key is to recognise this response and not to be afraid to accept that the stress response is an inbuilt warning system telling us that all is not well. By understanding what triggers work-related stress, we can be clear about the choices we make in responding to it. And although when experiencing stress it might not seem so at the time, we all have a choice about how we will deal with it. This includes our attitude towards the healing process and how we will move on from the negative effects of the experience. Would Marlborough or Disraeli have benefited from stress management techniques or the arsenal of medications available to today's stressed-out worker? It is questionable whether the outcome of their careers would have been affected, but such measures might have made their personal lives more bearable.

Who is susceptible?

Certain professions spring to mind as seeming more stressful than others: teachers, doctors, nurses, the police force, and any job having direct contact with the public. This preconception is actually backed up by a recent report on occupational stress which found that the groups in the UK who reported the highest levels of stress were indeed those in education and welfare professions such as teaching and nursing, as well as those in road transport and security.[9]

It has long been recognised that teachers are under enormous pressure to achieve national examination pass rate targets with dwindling resources. When questioned for the survey, two out of five in the teaching profession reported that they were experiencing high levels of stress. This is probably why the teaching profession actually has its own website, www.teacherstress.co.uk, which offers advice to teachers. An even worse profession for stress, according to a recent survey, is that of doctors, with an alarming four in five GPs reporting stress and overwork.[10] Indeed, researchers from University College London found after a 12-year study that nearly a quarter of all doctors are so stressed that they would be listed as psychiatric cases if they were to be seen by a mental health specialist.[11]

But teachers, doctors and policemen are not the only ones who suffer. The truth of the matter is that anyone, irrespective of age, gender or job description, can be susceptible to the negative effects of work-related stress. Any number of factors can cause work-related stress, as a report by academics at Bristol University concluded after a survey that investigated 17,000 randomly selected people from the Bristol electoral register. Their results showed that approximately 20% of the sample, in a wide variety of professions and pay scales, reported either high or extremely high levels of stress at work.[12]

This particular report concluded that various identifiable factors led to stress at work. It discovered, for example, that full-time employment incurred greater stress than part-time employment. Other factors causing work-related stress included job-overload, long hours, insufficient tools or support to do the job properly, bullying, short-term contracts, the threat of redundancy, and personal problems outside the workplace. No-one, it seems, is immune, especially since, as we shall see, many of these factors – such as bullying and heavy workloads – are becoming endemic in today's workplace.

The unhealthy workplace

What makes a workplace – and therefore its workers – healthy or unhealthy? A report by researchers at the University of Nottingham argues that work-related stress is caused primarily by the design and management of work environments and organisations. They accept that individual or personal factors are also possible causes but claim that organisations should promote, design and manage healthy work systems to prevent stress from developing.[13]

A healthy work place requires a balancing act. The Nottingham researchers found that to achieve a healthy work place, employees needed to be able to balance four aspects of work: (i) demand /pressure, (ii) knowledge, skills and abilities, (iii) a degree of control over working conditions, and (iv) support from others, whether co-workers or managers. When demands and resources are in balance, the work place can be described as healthy. Work-related stress is far more likely to occur if this balance is upset.

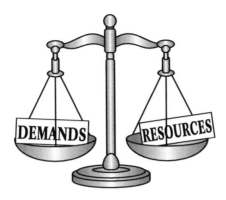

This model shows the ideal. But, as so many people in Britain know only too well, the ideal is often lamentably far from the real. Still, it is possible to bring the scales back into balance. But first, of course, we must know how we became unbalanced in the first place. Before turning to the cure for these problems, we must look more closely at the disease.

Work overload

Anxiety is the price we pay for civilization.

Sigmund Freud (1865-1939)

When we accept a job offer, we usually do so after reading through and agreeing to the job description with its lists of tasks expected to be performed. Many of us accept in trust that the job can be achieved within the contracted weekly working hours, which in most cases amount to 37 hours per week. Most of us also readily accept the miscellaneous clause in our job description that says we will 'undertake duties relevant to the post that might be in addition to one's usual duties'. Although worded in many different ways, this clause basically gives the employer the right, within reason, to ask us to do additional tasks on top of our job description.

So what is an acceptable additional task? This is where you need to ask some key questions about your organisation and take responsibility for your own well-being. To cover for a colleague for a few days while he/she is off with a minor short-term illness like a head cold is not unreasonable. But it is unacceptable for an employer to expect its staff to cover for long-term or continuous absence. The inevitable consequences of such action are resentment, exhaustion, anxiety and eventual ill health.

The researchers at Nottingham University discovered a direct link between job stress and a heavy workload that is characterised by long hours and constant deadlines. The consequences of this kind of heavy workload are illustrated in the case of Christine, a 29-year-old English Literature graduate who, after several years working on her local newspaper, began a new job in marketing at a university in the Midlands. It had been a positive career move for her and she was very excited about the change. However, within a few weeks of starting the job, Christine discovered that it was virtually impossible to manage her workload. 'The work was unrelenting,' she remembers. 'As soon as I finished one task there were ten more to complete, all with tight deadlines. I found myself covering the work of my two colleagues, who were both off sick, as well as my own, which was hectic enough in the first place.'

In Christine's case there were serious pre-existing problems in her office when she joined the organisation, but she only became aware of these a few weeks into her job. Two of her colleagues were repeatedly off on sick leave and she found that, in order to complete successfully her own tasks, somebody had to finish theirs. As there was no-one else around to cover, and as Christine was on probation, she automatically shouldered their work, fearing that her own work would suffer if she did not do so. She soon found herself spending long hours in the office, even refraining from taking a lunch break and often working until 7pm or coming in at weekends. Her social life came to a standstill and eventually, as we shall see, she fell ill under the enormous strain.

There is sometimes a fine line between genuinely wanting to be helpful to your employer in difficult times and being used and abused by that employer for short-term gain. As an employee, you must therefore use your judgement before the pattern is set and ask yourself the following questions:

My workplace?

1. Is my department under-staffed?
2. Is there a history of cuts?
3. Do I feel insecure in my job?
4. Am I expected to work long hours?
5. Are lunch hours or breaks frowned upon?
6. Do I feel pressurised to be seen to be achieving?
7. Am I expected to do tasks with no technical/IT back up?
8. Am I in a job where I am made to feel guilty that the client/some other person will suffer if I do not do something?

If, as in Christine's situation, the answer to most of these questions is yes, then you are working in an unhealthy environment. Unless something drastic happens to change the status quo, work related stress beckons. It is worth keeping in mind, in the midst of panics about deadlines and 12-hour days at the office, the words of Rudyard Kipling: 'More men are killed by overwork than the importance of this world justifies.'

Overloading an employee with too much work often goes hand-in-hand with the culture of working long hours. Many organisations have adopted such a culture not necessarily as a deliberate organisational mission but as a result of cost-cutting and down-sizing. But there are some companies that do expect their employees to work late and frown on staff who leave the office before 7-8pm. The National Employee Benchmarks Survey confirmed, after questioning 2,000 employees, more than half of the UK workforce feels under pressure to work long hours.[14] Furthermore, the Department of Trade and Industry (DTI) reported that one in six employees now works more than sixty hours a week. The DTI, in conjunction with the business magazine *Management Today*, commissioned the National Overtime Survey, which questioned 508 employees across five sectors of the UK workforce. 28% of the sample said they believe working long hours was essential to their progress within the company[15] – a worrying development, given the close link between long hours and occupational stress.

Interestingly, research from the International Stress Management Association uk (ISMA uk) and Royal Sun Alliance supports these perceptions.[16] 54% of respondents in the ISMA survey reported working more than five days a week, stating that they did so at the request of their employer – this despite the fact that the government has issued guidelines that no-one should work more than 48 hours a week, longer hours being deemed bad for an employee's health. Three out of five employees were not paid for their extra hours in the office: 78% of women and 54% of men.[17] *The Huddersfield Daily Examiner* reported in November 2003 that, according to a study by the TUC, almost 400,000 people in the Yorkshire region undertake unpaid overtime, the average worker logging more than seven-and-a-half hours a week in unremunerated labour. This means the average worker gives his or her employer an extra day of free labour every week! This same report stated that a staggering £23 billion unpaid overtime is undertaken nationally each year. According to the TUC, managers, professionals, office workers and machinery operators are most likely to do unpaid work.[18]

Employers may be getting free labour from many of their employees, but these savings are a false economy because working long hours is, ultimately, unproductive – bad for the health of the employee and, by extension, for the company. The research from the ISMA uk and Royal Sun Alliance showed that 72% of respondents get stressed from too much work and that 41% of these people say it is reducing their productivity.

50% of respondents say that working long hours is damaging their health, and 20% of people have sought medical help.[19] One in five employees has sought medical help because of poor physical or mental health developed courtesy of overwork. This state of affairs is surely not conducive to a happy and healthy workforce!

Professor Cary Cooper, the ISMA uk President and Deputy Vice Chancellor of the University of Manchester Institute of Science and Technology, says: 'Employers are always saying that people are their most valuable resource and it's time they stopped talking and did something about it.'[20] Carole Spiers, from the ISMA uk, adds: 'When you look at the figures in our latest survey, if we were talking about a flu epidemic rather than stress at work there would be a public outcry about the scale of the problem. But while given sufficient time, flu tends to go away of its own accord, stress at work certainly doesn't.'[21]

As we have seen, too much work and excessively long hours can trigger work-related stress in many people, especially if an employee feels this extra work is not appreciated. It is too easy for someone like Christine not to take responsibility for her working situation and to blame her employer without taking action. And it is far too easy for an employer to fail to alleviate Christine's situation by not dealing with the continuous sick leave of her colleagues. At the very least, cover should have been organised so that Christine could get her work done efficiently. Both employer and employee must take responsibility in helping each other to make their work environment a safe and comfortable place, as each is dependent on the other for their personal well-being.

'An ounce of prevention is better than a pound of cure', as the saying goes. So by asking yourself some searching questions, it might be possible to avoid the pitfalls of work-overload from the outset.

Am I overworked?

1. Give examples of work overload in your job.
2. Why do you think this is occurring? Are you under new management? Is there a culture of taking excessive sick leave in your office? Is your boss a workaholic? Are you a perfectionist?
3. Do you think the problem could be due to your own poor time management? If no, give concrete reasons why not.
4. Are you someone who finds difficulty in saying no? If yes, have you been offered any training in this?

Bullying

Some people might think of bullying as only a childhood phenomenon – a nasty confrontation set in a landscape of classrooms and playgrounds. But, regrettably, as many workers discover, bullying is equally prevalent – and equally unpleasant – in the work place. According to the Community Practitioners' and Health Visitors' Association, for example, one in three of the 563 people questioned in the NHS said they had to take time off work because of bullying. Half of the health visitors, school nurses and community nurses report having been bullied by their managers.[22] Bullying would seem to have reached virtually epidemic proportions.

The statistics are worrying because, in extreme cases, a victim of bullying can actually suffer the symptoms of post traumatic stress disorder (PTSD) – a condition more usually associated with battlefields and disasters than the office. Indeed, employees bullied by their co-workers are even more likely than air crash survivors and emergency services staff to suffer from PTSD: they rank only slightly lower than rape victims and those wounded in battle.[23]

What constitutes bullying in the workplace, and what are its causes? Tim Field, founder of Success Unlimited, an organization that offers online advice on bullying, defines it as occurring 'when one person, typically (but not necessarily) in a position of power, authority, trust, responsibility, management, etc, feels threatened by another person, usually (but not always) a subordinate who is displaying qualities of ability, popularity, knowledge, skill, strength, drive, determination, tenacity, success, etc. The bully has conditioned himself, or allowed himself to be conditioned, to believe that he can never have these qualities which he sees readily in others.'[24]

A bully can be someone who refuses to recognise another person's performance, loyalty and achievement, or it can be someone who is overly critical of a colleague, constantly humiliating or shouting at him. 'The full spectrum ranges from a person whose communication, interpersonal and behavioural skills are poor,' Field writes, 'to those who are spiteful, vindictive and destructive and who use their position of power to practise these traits for their own gratification.'[25]

Bullying is often difficult to prove. It can occur over long periods of time behind closed doors with no witnesses, and it can take very subtle – but no less damaging - forms. It can also be ignored by senior management, in a climate of cost-cutting and achieving all-important company targets, since it is the bully who can seem loyal to the company by visibly working long and unsociable hours. But this time commitment is, once again, a false economy. Companies must address the reason why an employee perceives himself or herself to have been bullied and then take constructive action.

Sally, a physiotherapist working in an NHS hospital in Bristol, might not at first blush seem like a typical victim of bullying. She had twelve years experience in three hospitals in Somerset before starting her present job, for which she was hired specifically because of her skills in working with trauma victims. Happily married with no children, she was passionate about her job but also enjoyed a healthy social life, including captaining the local ladies' hockey team, for which she played twice a week. Attractive, self-confident and popular, she did not regard herself as a candidate for bullying.

Problems arose, however, after one of her co-workers, Moira, was promoted internally after the existing manager took employment elsewhere. 'She seemed to change towards me overnight,' Sally explains. 'This was such a shock because when I first began work in the department, we often lunched together and met socially with our husbands. I considered her a friend, someone in whom I could confide.'

Sally's friendship with Moira dwindled rapidly. Little cliques soon formed in the office as Moira, who had received no management training, began to surround herself with people she liked and trusted. Sally, to her surprise, discovered she was not one of them. Moreover, she found herself the target of her new manager's somewhat threatening attentions. 'It was little things at first – making a note of my arrival and departure times, until she was actually checking up on me to see if I was at meetings I was supposed to attend. This baffled me,' Sally said, 'as the department worked on a trust system and I was always willing to cover for colleagues or work at weekends and evenings as we were sometimes asked to do.'

Sally was astonished how petty her manager suddenly became, listening to gossip and always taking the side of the person who passed it on. She soon found herself excluded from the information loop, and on many occasions she was the last to hear of office developments or hospital policies. She once turned up at a regional meeting of physiotherapists to discover that colleagues from other hospitals knew of funding made available for her physiotherapy department – a development that a shocked Sally knew nothing about. It was not long before she was regularly told that anonymous patients were 'complaining' to Moira about her supposedly rude or surly manner – something that had never happened in her previous jobs.

So why did Moira become a bully? And why did she single out Sally for her victim? Sally thinks, in retrospect, that it was largely the result of Moira feeling out of her depth as a manager. 'Moira had grave reservations at first about accepting the promotion,' Sally says. 'She used to claim that I was more qualified than she was, which in a way was true since I'd completed the Certificate and Diploma in Management Studies. After her promotion she seemed paranoid about me, as if she were worried that I was after her job. She seemed to want to discredit me, as if I were her competition rather than her co-worker. Anything I did or said was taken down and used against me. It was incredibly awful.'

Moira is, in many ways, a classic bully. Mary Sherry, an organisational psychologist from Asset Management Partnership, claims that in her experience women who feel out of their depth and who have no managerial training often become bullies. And female bullies, she feels, are more subtle than men in how they bully.[26] Dr Charlotte Raynor, from the Business School at Staffordshire University, agrees, adding that women are more likely than men to withhold information and isolate colleagues[27] – a divide and rule strategy that Moira deployed to devastating effect.

Anyone who has been on the receiving end of any form of bullying – from the playground to the boardroom - understands how totally devastating the experience can be. When it first started happening to her, Sally began questioning her own reactions to events, wondering if she was in fact being too sensitive or was interpreting things negatively. Soon, however, it became evident that she was not in fact being overly sensitive, and that both her work and self-confidence were being systematically undermined.

In an ideal world, a balanced and self-confident human being would be able to spot in the early stages of the bullying cycle that a problem is emerging. However, how many of us are truly balanced and completely self-confident? It is far easier to project such an image externally, especially one devised for the work place, than actually to be able to live it from our very core. Sadly, for most of us, by the time we realise we are being bullied it is too late. The damage has already begun to set in and, as our confidence begins to wane, we start to question our own abilities. 'I reached a very low ebb,' says Sally. 'All I knew is that I needed help – and fast.'

Part Two of this book will be particularly helpful in identifying who you should contact for advice and support if you are a victim of bullying. But first it might be useful to be clear in your own mind what is happening to you.

Am I the victim of a bully?

1. Why do you think you are a victim of bullying? List examples.
2. Who is bullying you? Is it one person or a team?
3. How long has this been occurring?
4. How does it make you feel? Write down separately your emotional, physical and behavioural reactions.
5. What have you done so far to alleviate the situation at work? Who have you talked to?
6. Have you done anything outside work to help you cope with this situation? Taken up a hobby, talked to a counsellor or doctor?
7. How, ideally, would you like the situation to be resolved?

In the wrong job

'True work is not a job that we do to make a living, survive and pay the bills,' writes Nick Williams, founder of the Heart at Work Project. 'True work is concerned with finding and expressing the best that is within us – our love, creativity, heart and spirit – and creating the money we need to pay the bills and to support our desired way of life as a by-product.'[28]

But true work, like true love, is hard to find. And bad jobs can be like bad relationships – we stay in them for the wrong reasons. How many of us have taken a short-term temporary job to earn money only to find that, after a few weeks of uninspiring work, it becomes hard to motivate ourselves to get to work on time? According to Williams, finding yourself in the wrong job can lead to depression and kill your creativity and passion. Or as Honoré de Balzac wrote, 'An unfulfilled vocation drains the colour from a man's entire existence.'

The experience of Steve, a 24-year-old university graduate, illustrates the difficulties of finding 'true work'. Working as a researcher for a local London council seemed a logical step for him at first, even though it was not his 'dream job'. Since his parents lived in London, he was able to stay at home while he found his feet financially, and began paying off several thousand pounds of student debts. After three years of independent living at university, Steve was not especially keen on moving back home to his parents, but financial circumstances and pressure from his family restricted his choice of jobs and locations. However, this compromise quickly proved a disaster.

'After nearly two years on the job, I felt like a zombie,' he says. 'There was no will power on the part of any of my colleagues to try anything different or make their jobs more interesting. I knew I had to get out, but the longer I stayed the more fearful I became of what I could do instead. I know this was stupid because the job was always going to be temporary until I paid off my student debts. But, in retrospect, it seemed that my job was killing my reason for being.'

Steve's situation is by no means unusual. The researchers at Nottingham University argue that career stagnation is certainly a hazardous condition of work[29]. But Steve's situation need not have become so dire. Had he made a clear plan at the beginning, this compromise may well have worked for him. Sometimes it is necessary for us to take the 'wrong job' initially in order to reach our long-term goal. So, despite his initial feeling at the interview that this job was not right for him, with the correct mindset Steve could have accepted this job as a kind of marriage of convenience, living at home for a short period while he cleared his debts and, in the meantime, gaining skills and experience before looking further afield for something more fulfilling. However, like many young graduates, Steve had no long-term objective and soon felt trapped. Because he had no idea about what he wanted to do with his life, he began to despair that his unfulfilling job was all that was on offer for him. 'I suppose my worst fear,' he said was, 'that I'd still be doing the same job at forty or fifty.'

It wasn't long before Steve started coming down with frequent head colds and persistent sore throats, which developed into a general feeling of malaise. More seriously, he also began to suffer from back pain, an affliction he had never previously experienced. Although Steve couldn't verbalise it, he was actually suffering from the stress of being in the wrong job, and this stress, besides making him ill, was drastically crippling his creativity and passion for life.

It is not unusual for us to enter the sort of compromise made by Steve, especially if the job offers financial security and material rewards that enable us to have a lifestyle we enjoy. But we can also stay in the wrong job through inertia. Change of any type can be scary, and the fear of change is enough to paralyse some people - we have all heard the saying, 'better the devil you know.' But it is a tremendous shame if we settle for less than we are worth, both in our jobs and in our personal lives. Because each of us, says Williams, has unique qualities and gifts, and finding our niche in our work can open up a whole spiritual dimension, enriching our lives and our relationships to work.

Am I in the wrong job?

1. What were your reasons for accepting your current job? Be completely honest, and be clear as to your motivation and long-term goals.
2. How long do you plan to stay in this particular job or profession?
3. Do you have a plan of action for the time you remain in this job, such as pursuing hobbies, re-skilling, taking courses?
4. Are you at a complete loss as to what to do next? If yes to this question, part two of this book will help you to identify who and what can assist you in your quest.

Job insecurity

It should come as no surprise to anyone that job insecurity – and the fear of redundancy and looming unemployment – is a great cause of stress. According to the *Bristol Stress and Health at Work Study*, respondents who were worried about losing their job ticked the box for high levels of stress.[30] John, a local authority careers officer in north-east England, experienced exactly this sort of insecurity when the careers service he was working for in the mid-1990's was subject to reorganisation. 'For eighteen months we had the threat of redundancies hanging over our heads. We didn't know how many jobs were to go, but our manager seemed to enjoy the insecurity and unhappiness we were all experiencing,' John explained. 'She even pitted us against each other, so in the end everyone was out only to save their own necks, even if it was at the expense of a colleague.'

The situation was made worse for John as he had recently taken out a mortgage with his fiancée and they were saving for their wedding, planned for the following year. They were even talking in the long-term of having children, but the threat of redundancy had put all this on hold and added pressure to the relationship. 'I began to worry,' says John, 'that I would lose my fiancée as well as my job.'

In Pete's case, job insecurity over a long period triggered both stress and depression. He was the IT manager in a large travel company that, in the economic downturn after 9/11, suffered severe financial problems. 'You should have seen my office,' he says. 'The stuffing was coming out of my chair and the office sofa had prolapsed. It was all a real mess.' He managed to survive several rounds of redundancies, even turning down, at one point, a healthy exit package. 'In retrospect I wish I'd had the courage to take them up on their initial offer. By the time I was finally forced to take redundancy, the company had gone bust and they could only afford to pay me the statutory minimum – not much after twenty years service with a staff of twenty-one under me. My bank account, not to mention my self-esteem, was severely compromised.'

The insecurity caused by the threat of redundancy can be exacerbated not only if the financial exit package is low or non-existent, as in Pete's case, but also if there is difficulty in finding new employment. However, although you might not be able to save your job, you can reduce the negative effects of redundancy by taking advice on when to bail out – if, like Pete, you have a choice – and by arming yourself with knowledge of the law, so that you know your rights. 'Forewarned is forearmed,' as the saying goes – and much of this ammunition will be found in Chapter Three.

Under the axe?

1. Is the threat of redundancy fact or fiction? If rumours are circulating, where are they coming from?
2. How much time have you left before redundancy kicks in?
3. Are you secretly pleased redundancy looms as you never liked your job or place of work? Be honest, because this might be a chance to change direction.
4. Do you feel devastated that you might be made redundant? If yes, ask yourself why? Is it based on financial reasons, or will you genuinely miss this job?
5. Will you look for a similar job elsewhere?
6. Are you planning to do something completely different like travel, re-train, or seek self-employment?

Part-time love?

Redundancy from a permanent job such as John or Pete's is difficult enough to face once or maybe twice in a career. But some people are confronted with this stress-inducing situation on a regular basis – for such is the plight of someone who works on short-term contracts.

For some, short-term contracts are a welcome way of life and fit in with their life-styles. However, for others, short-term contracts are the only way to get a foot in the door and because of the perpetual insecurity involved, can turn into a negative experience.

Thirty-eight-year-old Fay applied for a job in the archive department of a local council in Wiltshire at a time when there were only short-term contracts on offer. She was newly divorced and wished to live near to her parents in the West Country. She accepted a one-year contract, when offered, with the intention of making it permanent if at all possible. 'At first I didn't think about it, but about four months before the contract was to end I started to get anxious. I really didn't want to move. There were three of us in the same boat. I had so many sleepless nights assessing whether I should start applying for jobs in other areas.'

Fay and her two colleagues were eventually hired for another five years on one-year temporary contracts. As a result of the ongoing insecurity she suffered insomnia and bouts of stomach problems that always recurred a few months before each contract ended. 'As soon as my job was confirmed, these ailments would clear up,' she says. 'Until the next time, that is.'

Fay is one of many people in the UK who work – voluntarily or otherwise – on short-term contracts. According to a recent study by researchers at Birkbeck College, University of London, short-term and temporary contracts are on the increase in the UK. Between 1992 and 1996 those in temporary work rose by 30%, while fixed-term contracts rose by 25% and agency temping by 37%. More than half (57%) of UK firms use temporary workers, and 9.2% of the British workforce are temporary employees. So much, it seems, for the old idea of 'a job for life'.[31]

The Birkbeck researchers found that the reasons for the rise in temporary contracts were complex, varying from sector to sector and even within the departments of a single organisation. However, they concluded the rise had occurred for a number of reasons:

- the need to cut costs
- preparations for privatisation, sell-offs, de-mergers
- the need to concentrate on a company's core function while out-sourcing non-core activities
- legislation for compulsory competitive tendering and 'best value' in the public bodies
- pressures to develop internal markets[32]

The European Agency for Safety and Health, in its recent report, also found a rise in temporary contracts. In addition, they reported that a higher accident rate is documented for temporary workers, and that employees on temporary or fixed-term contracts have less access to training, less control over their working time, and fewer career prospects. These factors can obviously contribute to work-related stress.[33]

It seems that employers need to address some of these issues if they want to safeguard the health of their employees. But in an era of increasing short-term contracts, how can you reduce the negative side-effects of temporary work? First of all, ask yourself the questions at the end of this section in an attempt to determine what is behind your reservations about a temporary contract. Your financial situation usually plays an important role in your relationship to temporary work. However, once this is identified as a fear, it is easier to look at solutions, and these will be discussed in Chapter Five.

Am I happy with short-term contracts?

1. List the reasons why you are working on a short-term contract? Does this suit your lifestyle?
2. Do you feel you have no choice? If yes, list all the reasons why you think you have no choice.
3. Does working on short-term contracts make you feel insecure? Write down all the feelings you have.
4. What have you done so far to change the situation?
5. Write down all the positive things you can think of about working on a short-term contract.
6. What is your ideal solution? Don't hold back, because once you know exactly what you want the nearer you are to achieving it.

Personal problems: The 'home-work interface'

The only time we humans do not experience problems in our lives is, frankly, when we are dead. No life is free from peaks and troughs. Marriage, divorce, buying a house, the death of a loved one – all common experiences among workers of all ages – rate very highly on the stress scales, for obvious reasons. In 1967 two psychologists, T.H. Holmes and R.H. Rahe, devised a do-it-yourself stress test, the Holmes Stress Scale, that allows people to measure the impact of such events in terms of the probability of their leading to illnesses or accidents (see Appendix 1). Rating highest was the death of a spouse (100), followed by divorce (73) and marital separation (65). Work-related events scored lower: a change of job (36), a change of responsibility at work (29), trouble with the boss (23) and a change in working hours (20) were all rated as somewhat less stressful than, say, retirement (45) or pregnancy (40). However, stress is cumulative, and the Holmes Stress Scale aims to measure the impact of a number of events taken together. For example, a change of job combined with a marital separation and a new mortgage gives a person a 35% chance of suffering illness or an accident within two years. Anyone scoring over 300 on the test has, alarmingly, an 80% chance.

Holmes and Rahe argue that we should not try to avoid change; however, the body can only take so much 'social readjustment', and so much accompanying stress, at any one time, and therefore they advise that we budget in advance for any major life changes. Unfortunately, this planning is often easier said than done, as Joy, for example, discovered to her cost when two life-changing events unexpectedly occurred within a couple of months of each other.

Joy, 52, worked as a bank teller in a building society in Sheffield. She loved her job and had been with the company for seventeen years. She especially enjoyed working with the public and often received compliments from customers about her cheery and efficient manner.

Things at home, however, were not quite so satisfactory. Joy's mother had been terminally ill for nearly a year, which meant that most weekends, after working full time during the week, Joy would travel the two hundred miles round trip to help her father care for her mother, leaving her husband of twenty years at home to look after their teenage children.

As the weeks passed, Joy increasingly became more exhausted and short-tempered. There were frequent arguments with her husband, who started returning from work later and later each day, leaving her to sort out the household chores alone. Joy soon started suffering from insomnia, compounding her existing fatigue, and from uncontrollable crying in the privacy of her bedroom.

As stress gradually built up over the months, Joy was unaware how poorly she was coping, although she did recognise that she was tired and unhappy with her life. Still, she did not think this was a problem and assured herself it would eventually pass. When colleagues at work tried to help her, she shut them out, dismissing their concern as inappropriate. Matters drastically reached a head when Joy's husband left the marital home a week before Christmas, and she found herself with the sole responsibility of coping with her children whilst caring for her mother, who died less than a month later.

Matters at work came to a head three weeks after her mother's funeral when Joy became aggressive and angry with a customer – a woman with whom she had dealt successfully for many years - over a trivial misunderstanding. As she was being calmed with a cup of tea by her sympathetic but increasingly frustrated manager, Joy broke down and could not stop crying.

Joy's situation clearly illustrates how 'life's rich tapestry' – as our difficult experiences are bravely but euphemistically known - can cause stress that overflows into our working life. Customers who once gave Joy such pleasure had become a contributing cause of her stress. In Joy's case, an understanding manager prevented this temporary blip in her exemplary seventeen-year career from ruining her life. After four months off on sick leave, she was well enough to return to the job that she once so enjoyed.

Joy's story has a happy ending, but modern family life, in particular juggling children with work demands, has long been recognised as a trigger for stress. And no wonder, as we now find that an average working mum spends an additional two and a half hours per week in employment compared to the early 1990's. For working mothers with children aged between 12 –15 years, the figures are even higher, as they are likely to work five more hours a week than they did in the early 1990s.[34] In an interview broadcast on BBC Radio 4 in 2001, Shirley Conran, the author of *Superwoman*, advised women of childbearing age not to have children for the next ten years because of the lack of support for mothers. However, since that interview the government has ratified legislation in favour of parents by increasing and extending maternity leave and pay, and introducing rights to paid adoption and paternity leave. This is in addition to unpaid parental leave to care for a child under five, and unpaid time off work for any employee needing to deal with an emergency or unexpected situation involving a dependent such as an elderly parent.[35]

Offering more concessions to working parents is not the answer for lightening everyone's burden, however, as Ruth, a 43 year-old maternity nurse from Warwickshire, explains. Single with no children, Ruth finds that her personal life impacts on her working day in ways that increase her frustration. 'If my car breaks down, or the washing machine floods the kitchen, I still have to juggle getting these fixed within the constraints of my job,' she says. 'Unless you have an understanding boss, it can be days before it is possible to have the time to deal with domestic problems.'

Ruth argues that the stress single people have in juggling their lives with jobs, although different from that of parents, exists in other ways. According to the 2001 census of England and Wales, over 30% of the adult population is single (never-married). In addition, separated or divorced adults make up 10.6% of the population, while 8.4% of adults are widowed and, in many cases, also living alone.[36] These figures, taken together, mean that potentially 49% of the adult population, many of whom are in the work force, live alone. In 1971 by contrast, only 18% of adults lived alone![37]

'I'm not against flexible working conditions,' says Ruth 'but it has to be inclusive for everyone. In my experience it is the worker with young children who gets first option on flexible working. And in reality this means I am the one who tends to do the night shifts and the public holidays, and I feel not only is this unfair, but it sometimes adds to my personal stress. I never seem to have time to catch my breath even when I do get my couple of weeks' annual leave.'

Ruth has been fortunate: the stresses from her personal life, combined with a busy career, have so far not affected her health. But not everyone is so lucky with their work: Sally, Fay and Christine, along with many thousands of other British workers, have been made so unwell by their jobs that they require medical help for a wide constellation of symptoms and illnesses, often very serious. The next chapter will take a closer look at the debilitating physical and mental effects of work-related stress. In the meantime, it might be helpful to identify if personal problems are affecting your work.

Are personal problems affecting my work?

1. Are you experiencing a major event in your life? What is it – marriage, death, divorce, moving house, unemployment, illness?
2. Refer to Appendix 1, the Holmes Stress Scale, and add up the Life Changes you have experienced in a year.
3. Do you feel more than usually frustrated or unhappy with your life? If yes, list the things that particularly irritate or bother you. Be completely honest even if it seems trivial.
4. Think back to a happy event in your life and write down why it makes you happy? What are you feeling? What were the circumstances? Why is your life so different now?
5. Do you have a support network you can tap into – friends, advice help lines, family who listen, work colleagues? If yes, how do you think they have helped you?
6. Ideally, how would you like your personal problem to be solved?
7. In your words, why do you think this is not possible?

2 BODIES, BRAINS AND STRESS

It is health that is real wealth and not pieces of gold and silver.

Mohandas Gandhi

The power of love is now something, it seems, that scientists celebrate as much as poets and songwriters. Studies have shown that patients who feel loved can make remarkable recoveries from serious illnesses, often against incredible odds. Dr Dean Ornish, the founder of the Preventative Medicine Research Institute in California, has for over twenty years been conducting research into reversing severe coronary heart disease by making life-style changes in his patients. He found that out of 159 people undergoing coronary angiography, those suffering from the fewest blockages in their arteries were the ones who felt the most loved and supported.[1] Another study discovered that patients who felt the most isolated had almost four times the risk of dying prematurely.[2] In still another study, the late Dr David McClelland, a renowned psychologist at Harvard University, showed that the production of salivary antibodies to fight infection were increased when a group of students were shown a film of Mother Theresa comforting a child. These same antibodies became depressed when the students then watched scenes of war.[3]

As this research indicates, our physical state depends very much on our mental state. Dr McClelland's work proves that feelings of love can stimulate our immune system, and it is our immune system, of course, that helps protect us against viruses and infections. Someone suffering from work-related stress is probably not feeling particularly beloved, to say the least. Hence, this natural phenomenon – an immune response triggered by feelings of love – might be temporarily switched off, leaving sufferers from stress more vulnerable to illnesses.

A body on a high state of stress alert, as we have seen in the previous chapter, can change physically: Sally, Steve, Christine and Fay – all fell ill under the pressures of work. Being in a state of stress for prolonged periods can trigger, in some people, a host of ailments, including emotional, behavioural and psychological problems, all of which are urgent warning signs requiring swift attention.

The Physical Symptoms

'I was tired all of the time,' Sally remembers. 'No matter how early I went to bed I'd wake up feeling completely exhausted. The doctor gave me tests for glandular fever, iron deficiency, thyroid problems and diabetes. It got to the point where I was desperately hoping that they would discover a root physical cause for my tiredness, no matter how horrible. But nothing showed up.'

One of the first signs of stress – and an early signal that all is not well – is fatigue. As we have seen, Sally was bullied on and off for over eighteen months. After the first few months, she started experiencing extreme lethargy. She continually felt that she was coming down with the flu or worse, but nothing definite ever materialised. According to Dr Christiane Northrup, an obstetrician and gynaecologist, fatigue can be the result of 'unabated stress over long periods of time in the face of insufficient nutrients in the diet.' All this can lead, she writes, to adrenal exhaustion. The adrenal glands are extremely important in the body, as they secrete the key hormones that are essential in getting us through the day with energy, enthusiasm and efficiency. If these become depleted, fatigue is inevitable.[4]

Besides fatigue, Sally also developed tension headaches that often struck during work and lasted for several hours. After about a year of all these symptoms, she began suffering back and neck pains, a common symptom caused by muscles tensed due to the stress response. In addition she became tearful and would overreact to the smallest upset, and occasionally she even experienced heart palpitations – a symptom which she found extremely alarming. When she began having trouble sleeping she found herself physically at her lowest ebb and began to feel depressed.

Report after report links stress to illness. Stress has been associated with peptic ulcers, for example, because the stomach produces more acid in response to stressful situations. Increases in blood pressure, heart diseases and strokes are also related to stress, as researchers found at a hospital in France. They studied the blood pressure in over 300 workers in a chemical factory. All the workers were healthy at the time of the research and aged between 18-55 years. 20% of the subjects reported that they perceived a high level of job strain, and interestingly enough, the same 20% showed higher blood pressure levels than their co-workers when they were all measured at a later date.[5]

High blood pressure can lead to strokes and heart attacks. Researchers at the University of Michigan, along with colleagues in Finland, studied the blood pressure responses to a stressful situation of over 2,300 men in eastern Finland. Over the course of 11 years they found that the men who had exaggerated blood pressure rises in response to stress had a 72% greater risk of developing a stroke than those who didn't react so strongly to stress.[6]

Charles was extremely lucky that his heart attack, caused in large part by the stress of his job, did not kill him. A managing director of an international company, he collapsed at work one day with severe, debilitating chest pains. Charles, 54, remembers how prior to his collapse he felt extremely overwrought. In addition to working as one of the company's managing directors, he negotiated the buying of smaller companies, frequently travelling all over the world. He regularly worked a fourteen-hour day, which he didn't mind since he loved the work so much. When his wife begged him to slow down, he simply ignored her.

What seemed to have tipped the balance for Charles was being given an additional task. 'We realised that many of our senior staff were of retirement age and there was no-one to fill their shoes,' he explained. 'I was asked to take charge of this.' This meant that, on top of working a fourteen-hour day, Charles was forced to take work home at weekends to cover this additional workload. In the previous twelve months, he had only taken one week of vacation, leaving his body completely exhausted.

Not only is stress a culprit in causing rising blood pressure; it is also linked to health problems created by cortisol, the 'stress hormone', which is released by a body under pressure. This hormone is not just a marker for stress levels: it is vital for the functioning of almost every part of the body. Excesses or deficiencies of cortisol can lead to 'dis-ease'.

HOW CORTISOL WORKS

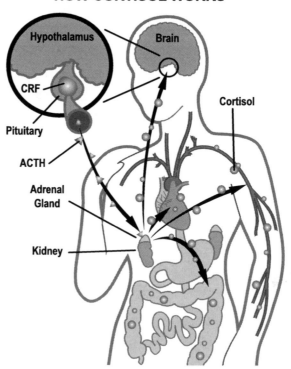

So what is cortisol? Cortisol is a hormone secreted by the adrenal glands, which are found near the kidneys. When not produced by stressful events, cortisol plays an important role in the regulation of blood pressure, of cardiovascular function, and of the body's use of proteins, carbohydrates, and fats. But any stress experienced by the body, whether physical (illness, trauma, surgery, extremes of temperature) or psychological, results in increased cortisol secretion. A chain reaction of events then occurs whereby the blood sugar rises so the brain will have more energy-giving glucose. Remember the 'fight or flight' scenario? At the same time that the brain receives more glucose, the other tissues of the body correspondingly decrease their use of glucose as fuel. The body therefore becomes sluggish and does not work to its full capacity. In other words, the normal functioning of the body tips out of balance. All of this explains why *prolonged* stress can be harmful to your health. It can disturb the hormone balance, and the knock-on effect could be an under-active thyroid gland, which can lead to weight gain, fatigue and sluggishness.[7]

Stress can also produce other, possibly unexpected, symptoms. 'I had never suffered from PMS before,' says Christine. 'But during my "Inferno year", as I call it, I suddenly started having PMS and bad periods. We're talking pain, bloating, acne, mood swings – all the textbook stuff. It was just one more thing to worry about. I kept wondering, "Why now? Why this on top of everything else?"'

In fact, there's probably a biological reason why Christine began experiencing menstrual problems at a time of stress. Researchers from the University of Cincinnati found that stress was associated with various menstrual disorders. Interviews with 170 healthy, pre-menopausal women in the U.S. Air Force found that those women who reported higher levels of life event stresses had an increased incident of dysmenorrhoea (severe pain during menstruation), hypermenorrhea (heavy bleeding) and abnormal menstrual cycle length.[8] One recent study has suggested that stress has an effect on women's ability to conceive, since high levels of cortisol were found in women who did not have periods or suffered irregular ones.[9] Cortisol can also increase the production of oestrogen. Secreted by the ovaries, oestrogen and progesterone are commonly known as the 'female hormones'. The properties of each offset the other, and too much of one – in this case oestrogen – can cause PMS, endometriosis, ovarian cysts, fibroids and menopausal problems. Oestrogen regulates the menstrual cycle, lifts our mood and acts as a growth hormone for the breast, uterine and ovarian tissue when producing babies. However, too much oestrogen can cause breast stimulation that can lead to fibrocystic breast or breast cancer. Researchers in Finland discovered, for example, that stressful life events may increase a woman's risk of developing breast cancer because of the increase of cortisol.[10]

As if all of this were not enough, yet another alarming effect of increased cortisol secretions has been studied by Dr Bruce McEwen at Rockefeller University in New York. Dr McEwen has found that long-term stress can actually lead to mental impairment due to the fact that cortisol 'remodels' the hippocampal region of the brain – the part of the brain, that is, that deals with memory.[11]

As this wealth of research indicates, people suffering from stress can experience a wide constellation of physical symptoms. Many of these problems can be successfully treated with medication; others, however, are much more difficult and dangerous, as we shall see in the next section. Listed below are some common symptoms of the effects of stress.

- Fatigue
- Trembling
- Headaches and migraines
- Nausea or vomiting
- Frequent colds and sore throats
- Abdominal cramps
- Heart palpitations
- Diarrhoea
- Chest pains
- Stiff neck or muscles
- Insomnia
- Back pain
- High blood pressure
- Flushing or sweating
- Loss of appetite
- Feeling cold
- Abnormal thirst
- Physical numbness (toes, fingers, lips)
- Shingles
- Irritable bowel syndrome
- Skin disorders (athletes foot, eczema, psoriasis, shingles, ulcers)
- Hormonal problems (disturbed menstrual cycle, loss of libido, impotence)

Source: **www.teacherstress.co.uk**

The Psychological Symptoms

It is not just the body that suffers under stress. Work-related stress may also affect the mind. In extreme cases, usually identified with bullying or harassment, an individual can experience the symptoms of post traumatic stress disorder, such as flashbacks, nightmares, phobias, detachment, paranoia and severe aversion to the causes of the stress.[12] Other psychological symptoms experienced by those suffering from job stress, such as depression, are more common but no less debilitating, as Joy was to discover. For the first two weeks that she was signed off work by her doctor, she found that she would sit on the sofa for hours on end, staring blankly at the TV screen or into her garden. She felt so depressed that even the effort of making her lunch proved an enormous task. 'I would keep obsessing about that last day when I rowed with a customer at the building society,' she explains. 'I could still feel everyone looking at me as if I was mad. I felt so ashamed, and then I would cry for what seemed like hours. This went on for weeks.'

Bereavement, divorce, losing a job or other personal tragedies are all common experiences that most of us must go through at some stage of our lives. Feeling depressed or 'blue' is also a common reaction to such experiences. Most people, after a few weeks, will return to their normal state of affairs. However, if the feelings of sadness or hopelessness last for longer, clinical depression may be indicated. Some statistics show that at least one in four people will experience mental health problems, such as depression, that require some sort of assistance.

Depression is a complex condition. It occurs as a result of abnormalities of certain chemicals in the brain. These chemicals are called neurotransmitters, which are secreted by the brain and nervous system. To date 60 have been discovered with yet more to be identified. Researchers have found that people with depression have lower levels of the chemical produced in the brain called serotonin. This chemical has a powerful effect on our mood, influencing our perception of pain, our sleep, our appetite and even our motivation. Besides affecting blood pressure and the menstrual cycle, cortisol in excess levels can also inhibit the production of serotonin.[13]

In other words, if you are suffering from work-related stress, there could be a biological reason why you are also experiencing depression, since difficult life events can cause neurotransmitters to become unbalanced. A person suffering from depression might unwittingly make his situation worse by relying too much on alcohol in an attempt to feel better and then developing a poor diet, thus leaving himself vitamin deficient – and too much alcohol and too little vitamin B-12 and folic acid are also linked to depression. The correct workings of the body are therefore reliant on the whole body – the mental and the physical – being in perfect harmony.

Depression brings with it another problem. Saying you're depressed is not quite like saying you have the flu, or a heart condition. As one study of stress puts it: 'Mental illness carries with it a stigma that is not attached to those who suffer from demonstrably physical conditions.'[14]

Christine discovered, to her horror, that not everyone – including family and close friends – understood or appreciated her diagnosis of depression. 'Explaining to people that I was off work with depression and work-related stress was a nightmare,' she says. '"But you look so well" was often the reply. Then I felt I had to justify and explain what I'd been through, and it all sounded so silly. On many occasions I wished I had a broken leg or something so they could accept why I was off sick.'

If you are experiencing any of the symptoms below then you might be suffering from depression, a possible result of stress. It is advisable to consult your doctor.[15]

- More often than not, I am depressed for most of the day
- I have lost my enthusiasm for most activities
- I have problems sleeping (insomnia, early morning wakening, excess sleep)
- I feel tired or fatigued for most of the time
- I have a low opinion of myself. I usually feel worthless or guilty
- I am unable to concentrate; I am indecisive
- I feel overwhelmed; I feel a sense of hopelessness
- I feel either edgy or slowed down
- I have suicidal thoughts. I don't want to be here anymore
- I have had a significant weight gain/loss not due to dieting

* * * *

In 1977 the Australian actor Peter Finch was posthumously given an Academy Award for his portrayal of disgruntled news anchorman Howard Beale in Sidney Lumet's satirical film *Network* (1976). Learning that he is to be fired by his television network after decades of service, Beale threatens to commit suicide on air, causing ratings to shoot up dramatically. Beale also creates a sensation by urging all of his listeners who are fed up with their jobs to stick their heads out of their office windows and shout what became – in both the movie and real life – a sort of war cry for the occupationally disenchanted: 'I'm mad as hell and I'm not going to take this anymore!'

Finch's Howard Beale is an extreme example of what might be called 'job rage'. People react differently to the emotional fallout from stress, but anger, either suppressed or openly expressed, can be a common reaction. In the months preceding his heart attack, Charles admitted to feeling irritable to such an extent that very little things would upset him. 'I seemed to be on a short fuse all of the time,' Charles, a managing director, explained. 'I recall shouting at my secretary one day when she spilt some coffee on my office carpet. She had been with me for years and we usually got on like the proverbial house on fire. But I hadn't asked her for a cup of coffee in the first place, so I threw a real wobbly, even though I didn't give a shit about the carpet or the coffee. Of course it didn't occur to me at the time that she had brought the coffee in to me because she was actually worried I was working too hard without a break.'

After giving him a piece of her mind, telling him he had been rude and aggressive for months, Charles's secretary stomped out of the office and took the rest of day off. Charles was furious. 'I could feel my blood boiling when I found out she had left the building as she was leaving me in the lurch - all over a spilt cup of coffee!'

What Charles did not realise at the time was that anger, like other emotions, is accompanied by physiological and biological changes: your heart rate and blood pressure go up, as do the levels of your energy hormones, adrenaline and noradrenaline. Anger is a natural response to threats; it prepares us to defend ourselves when attacked. In other words, a certain amount of anger, like stress, is necessary for our survival; too much, however, can be dangerous.

For Charles, anger in these circumstances was an unnecessary and unproductive response. But his body was already on 'high stress alert' as, after months of unrelenting work overload, he had unwittingly flooded his body with the hormone cortisol. Worryingly for Charles, his stress and anger were putting him at risk of serious health problems, since researchers have found that one of the most important variables in coronary heart disease is anger, and anger goes hand in hand with projections of hostility.[16]

Charles gave way to an uncontrollable burst of temper. But studies have shown that suppressing the anger is not the answer either, since this can be detrimental to your well-being. Research proves that people who suppress anger have a higher mortality rate over time, particularly in the case of women.[17] So if studies prove that expressing anger like Charles did is unhealthy, and suppressing anger is equally unhealthy, what are you to do? One suggestion might be anger management, which will be covered in more detail in Chapter Seven. In the meantime, try answering some of the following questions to determine whether anger management might help you.

Mad as hell?

1. Am I volatile by nature?
2. Have I ever been described as aggressive? If yes, do you think this was justified?
3. Have I noticed a change recently in my reaction to the behaviour of others?
4. Do I feel people generally let me down? If yes, how does that make me feel?
5. Am I someone who speaks before thinking?
6. Is everyone out to 'get me' so that I must never let my guard down? What are the reasons behind this thought pattern?
7. Give an example of someone or something that has made you feel very angry? How did you respond? How do you think you could have dealt with the situation better?

'Panic'

We have already seen how the 'fight or flight' reflex, first triggered in our prehistoric ancestors by woolly mammoths and sabre-tooth tigers, still arises in us when we feel threatened by someone or something. But what if someone experiences these heart-thumping, palm-sweating symptoms for no apparent reason – and in the unlikeliest of locations: the pet food aisle of the supermarket?

The uncertainty of one-year, short-term contracts certainly made Fay feel anxious and apprehensive about the future, so much so that she developed what is known as a panic disorder. 'I know the attacks must have been related to the stress of my contract coming to an end because they always occurred a month or two before my job was to finish,' she explained. Fay found that they would come on in the most unexpected places. 'I remember one time being in the pet food aisle of the supermarket and my heart started pounding as if I were running a marathon. I was so scared – I really thought that I was having a heart attack. I was hyperventilating and clinging on to the shopping trolley for dear life. No-one around me seemed to have noticed anything was wrong.'

According to the American Psychological Association, a panic attack 'is a sudden surge of overwhelming fear that comes without warning and without any obvious reason. It is far more intense than the feeling of being "stressed out" that most people experience.' You should always visit your doctor if you have a panic attack, as many of the symptoms that occur during an attack are the same as symptoms of diseases of the heart, lungs, intestines or nervous system. A doctor will be able to rule these out.

Panic attacks usually have both physical and psychological causes. Studies with twins have confirmed the possibility of 'genetic inheritance' of the disorder, but it could also be caused by a biological malfunction. Research in this area is ongoing. Panic attacks can usually be treated successfully, as we will see in more detail in Chapter Six. Symptoms of a panic attack include:

- racing heartbeat
- difficulty in breathing, feeling as though you 'can't get enough air'
- terror that is almost paralysing
- dizziness, light-headedness or nausea
- trembling, sweating, shaking
- choking, chest pains
- hot flushes or sudden chills
- tingling in fingers or toes ('pins and needles')
- fear that you're going to go crazy or are about to die[18]

Depression, anger and panic attacks are not the only psychological symptoms experienced from work-related stress. Below are some other common problems that can be triggered by stress.

- Poor concentration
- Anxiety
- Nervousness
- Frustration
- Worry

- Fear
- Irritability
- Impatience
- Indecisiveness
- Flashbacks and replays
- Excessive guilt
- Forgetfulness and poor memory
- Insecurity
- Desperation
- Feeling of isolation
- Disbelief and bewilderment

Source: **www.teacherstress.co.uk**

The Behavioural Symptoms

'I'd been brought up to believe that men don't cry. You know, stiff upper lip and all that,' says Mark, a 49-year-old deputy manager of a large retail store. 'But then I had a particularly bad day in the office when my manager had humiliated me once again in front of a senior manager. I was so shocked she had outright lied, I just stood there and said nothing. At home that night I had a blazing row with my wife. Then I stormed off to our games room and went over the day's events in my head again and again, until out of sheer frustration I broke down and sobbed.'

Too much stress causes our personalities to change along with our bodies. People act out of character: calm people become angry and impatient; cheerful people become sullen and withdrawn; natural leaders become indecisive and hesitant. Odd habits manifest themselves – grinding teeth, pacing, scratching. Tearfulness and irritability are often indicators, especially if they continue over long periods.

As work-related stress may build up over a period of time, it is often relatives who first notice differences in behaviour. 'My husband didn't say anything to begin with,' says Sally, 'but he noticed my mood constantly changing, from one minute being high as a kite and enthusiastic about changing my work situation, to being completely depressed and flat the next. He said it was almost as if I was on drugs, one that picked me up, another that completely laid me out.'

Hypervigilance is a common symptom of stress too, especially in cases of bullying. When people are constantly criticised in areas of their work, they soon start looking over their shoulders, trying to anticipate potential problems. Sometimes they are so hypervigilant that they see problems arising that not even the bully has perceived, as Mark discovered. 'I was constantly checking and re-checking my work – almost obsessively – to make sure I had not made any errors that she could use against me. I even made sure in advance that when I wanted to take leave, other staff would be in to cover so she couldn't deny my leave on those grounds. Looking back, it took so much of my time and energy just to try and stay one step ahead of my manager that I think how wasteful it all was, in terms of my productivity.'

Loss of a sense of humour and withdrawal from normal social activities are likewise common symptoms of stress. Christine had enjoyed the company of her friends on weekends. She used to go rambling with them several times a month, followed by lunch in a country pub. But soon she began making excuses and staying home. She also attended sculpture class once a week but withdrew from that as well. 'I just didn't have the heart for it anymore,' she explains. 'I didn't feel I could enjoy myself and ended up watching television in my flat or just pacing up and down the corridor, wearing out the carpet.'

After a while, Steve, too, did not wish to socialise. 'The last thing I wanted to do after a boring day in the office was play tennis. I'd always been a keen tennis player and as soon as I moved back home to my parents, I joined the local club. It was good for a while and I made some nice friends, but the more frustrated I became with work and my colleagues, the more I lost the will to do anything.' Steve let his tennis membership lapse while his racket gathered dust in a closet.

Besides stopping doing things that are good for us, like exercising and socialising, we can also, when under stress, start doing things that are bad for us. It is not uncommon for someone suffering from work-related stress to become more reliant on tea, coffee, alcohol, cigarettes or sleeping tablets. A cup of coffee with a cigarette, for example, seems like a calming break in a stressful day, but these drugs – nicotine and caffeine - can actually exacerbate our symptoms. It becomes a vicious cycle.

Judith, a deputy manager of a nursing home in Sussex, fell into exactly this sort of cycle. 'I've always been partial to a cup of coffee,' she explained, 'but my intake rose from about three or four cups a day to ten or eleven. My friends joked that I was a "coffeeholic" who kept the economies of several small coffee-producing nations afloat. It started off as a soothing drink when my manager was being exceptionally unreasonable, until I found that whenever I felt tired or harassed, I'd reach for the coffee pot or pop out to Starbucks.'

Judith soon found she was also drinking large amounts of coffee at home in the evenings and at weekends but couldn't at the time see any connection between her copious coffee intake and her insomnia. To make matters worse, her mugs of coffee were often enjoyed with chocolate bars. 'I'd always feel perked up after a bar of chocolate or a chockie biscuit,' she explained. What Judith did not realise is that caffeine is found not only in coffee but also in chocolate, tea, cola and certain over-the-counter medications.

How can caffeine cause anxiety, insomnia or even depression? Caffeine is a chemical that can interfere with our brain chemistry, making us feel more stressed – ready for action – because it provokes the release of excess stress hormones via its stimulant effects on the adrenal glands. It also interferes with a tranquillising neurotransmitter chemical in the brain called adenosine. Adenosine is the chemical that is released to switch off our anxiety levels in the 'fight or flight' reaction once the threat has disappeared. Caffeine can actually hinder the function of adenosine, so if you are already full of adrenaline, caffeine will exacerbate stress levels and anxiety by increasing the time it takes for your body to return to 'normal'.

Caffeine can also cause other troubles. It is a diuretic and can cause depletion of nutrients such as vitamin B6, which is involved in the manufacture of serotonin. As we have seen already, serotonin plays a powerful role in uplifting our mood. In addition, tea and coffee contain tannins. Tannins are plant polyphenols that occur naturally in tea leaves, bark, coffee beans, grapes, roots and resins, binding and precipitating proteins. They are what turn autumn leaves crimson, animal hides into leather, and your teeth – if you drink lots of tea – a dull yellow. But tannin in tea and coffee does something more, for it interferes with nutrient absorption of essential minerals including calcium, magnesium and the B vitamins. Tolerance for caffeine varies from person to person. If you think you need to cut your intake of caffeine, do this gradually over a number of weeks. Sudden withdrawal can cause uncomfortable side effects such as headaches. For every cup of tea or coffee, you should drink at least one glass of water to help flush the toxins through your kidneys and compensate for the diuretic effects of caffeine.

Am I a caffeine addict?

1. How many of the following do I consume each day?
   - cups of tea
   - cups of coffee
   - chocolate products
   - cola
2. Have I been consuming more of these products recently? If yes, when did I start this?
3. How do I feel immediately after I consume a caffeine product?
4. Do I suffer from any of the listed health problems below? If yes, caffeine might be aggravating the symptoms.

irritability	insomnia	depression
anxiety	osteoporosis	migraine
gastritis	panic	reduced fertility
palpitations	diabetes	PMS
hiatus hernia	tinnitus	indigestion

anaemia	fatigue	increased heart rate
raised blood		irritable bowel
pressure		syndrome

5. How many glasses of water do I drink a day?

* * * *

Not all insomnia can be eliminated along with the cups of coffee or bars of chocolate. Most sufferers of work-related stress will experience sleepless nights at some point. Learning to relax and shut out the day's distressing events is one of the hardest things to do: most of us have at one time or another spent the early hours of the morning lying awake, mulling over problems. Researchers at the University of Bristol found that very few highly stressed people said they were able to 'switch off' and relax when they came home from work.[19] Researchers at the Karolinska Institute in Stockholm found, after interviewing 5,700 employed men and women, those who spent their free time worrying about their jobs were more likely to suffer from sleep problems.[20] Interestingly, a report by Demos claims that the average Briton has accumulated a 'sleep deficit' of 25-30 hours. Their report says that lack of rest hurts the creativity and productivity of workers, as well as relationships at home. They suggest banning breakfast meetings and promoting siestas and 'sleep days' to allow weary staff to catch up on sleep.[21]

Pete, an IT project manager with a staff of 21 under him, suffered chronic insomnia as he dodged round after round of redundancies for over five years. 'After the second round of job losses my role literally disappeared, so I found myself being shunted around the company doing jobs I was not often qualified to do. I became the general dogsbody,' he explained. 'I didn't even have a desk and it made me feel so worthless. At night I could not get to sleep as I went over in my mind how unjust the situation was. How could a company I had worked for since I was eighteen treat me in such a way?'

Mark, a deputy retail manager, also found getting a good night sleep difficult during the time he suffered from work-related stress. 'If only I could get to sleep,' he said, 'I felt I would have been able to cope with my manager. Tiredness numbed my reactions and I started making mistakes – exactly what she wanted. Each mistake and each confrontation made it all the harder to sleep. I was trapped in a vicious circle.'

The link between daytime stress and restless sleep is well established, but what actually occurs in the body to cause insomnia? Researchers at the Sleep Research and Treatment Centre of the Pennsylvania State University College of Medicine found that people suffering from chronic insomnia have increased levels of stress hormones such as cortisol in the blood stream. When cortisol is activated, the body is ready for action and therefore, obviously, not ready for a peaceful night's sleep.[22] Pete and Mark, already suffering from work-related stress, found themselves in a state of hyperarousal in which the stress response could not be switched off along with the bedside lamp. Hence physically it was difficult for their bodies to relax enough to sleep well. But fortunately for Mark and Pete – and for any one else suffering from work-induced insomnia – there are any number of ways, as we shall see, to break this damaging cycle.

Listed below are further common behavioural symptoms that occur when we suffer from work-related stress:

- Tearfulness
- Throwing or hitting things
- Blaming
- Yelling
- Irritability
- Obsessiveness (talking about the experience)
- Sullenness
- Indecision
- Loss of sense of humour
- Pacing
- Fidgeting
- Nervous habits (nail biting, foot tapping)
- Picking
- Scratching
- Teeth grinding
- Comfort spending
- Shattered self confidence and self esteem

Source: **www.teacherstress.co.uk**

Stress and Relationships

Each has his past shut in him like the leaves of a book known to him by heart and his friends can only read the title.

Virginia Woolf

When examining how stress affects people, we often forget to mention an important group: the families, spouses and friends of the sufferers. They too can feel the effects, since the person they know and love can often change, as we have just seen, into someone quite different from his or her normal self.

Spouses in particular can experience their own anxiety about the situation. Often they feel powerless as their partner's personality and behaviour changes and they are forced to watch them decline physically and mentally. If they are in a relationship where problems are shared, the partner will hear story after story of injustice, or negative accounts of incidents from the office. Feelings of anger and helplessness are common among spouses. It is not long before the atmosphere of the whole household is infected with negativity – hardly the recipe for a relaxed and happy domestic life.

Likewise, it is not uncommon for spouses and children in the household to experience ill health. Judith, a 53-year-old care-worker from Kent, thinks that both her husband suddenly suffering from shingles and her daughter developing eczema were due to stress that built up in the household when she was being bullied by her manager in the nursing home. 'I can't prove it,' she says, 'but it just seems too coincidental that my husband and daughter, who never suffered from these ailments before, suddenly developed them during that stressful period. As a family we never hid any problems from each other or the children, so all of us were party to my unhappiness.'

Levels of stress in the household can be just as high if a person hides his work situation from a partner. 'I didn't think it was fair to dump my problems at work on my wife,' Mark explains. 'And also, I suppose there was a degree of male pride. Being bullied by a female boss younger than me just wasn't the kind of thing I wanted to tell my wife about.'

Mark was so badly affected by his treatment from his colleague at work that he became withdrawn and moody at home. So uncommunicative and uncaring did he become, in fact, that his wife of twenty-one years suspected him of conducting an affair. Tension in the household eventually got to the point where she threatened to leave him if they didn't go to Relate, the marriage guidance service, to sort out their problems. It was at the first session that Mark broke down and admitted everything he had been going through – and that the 'other woman' was actually his bullying manager. His relationship did not collapse, as he feared would happen, and his wife supported him in every way she could – an experience that Mark now thinks actually strengthened their marriage.

It is not just husbands and wives who bear the brunt. Margaret, a divorced 56-year-old, lived alone when she was bullied in a university library, and felt she could not unload her problems on her grown-up son, who lived in London. 'He was so worried by the tone in my voice that he came to visit me as soon as he could,' she remembers. 'He was visibly shocked by my appearance. After making me tell him what was going on – this was nearly a year after it began – he immediately wanted to help me. I still don't know how I would have written the official letters of complaint without him.'

Sometimes, however, the advice of well meaning friends or family can add to a sufferer's anxiety, as Sally discovered after confiding in some of her closest companions: 'Three people on separate occasions said to me it was outrageous how I was being treated. They all insisted I must stand up to my boss and just go in and do my job. But until you've experienced what it is like to be excluded and undermined over a long period of time, you have no idea how it affects your confidence, or for that matter, the will-power to change it. I felt they just didn't understand what I was going through.'

Sally suffered tremendous feelings of guilt when people told her that, if she didn't 'stand up for herself', her bullying manager would only victimize someone else in the future. She became so ashamed of her own 'weakness' – as her friends seemed to regard it – that she stopped seeing them socially.

Christine experienced a similar lack of sympathy and support when she discussed her problems with her father. He was mortified when he heard she had been given three months off on sick leave due to work-related stress. 'He had always been so supportive and I know he meant well, but he told me over and over I mustn't take sick leave for stress as it would be on my record and I'd never be promoted. Actually, he was wrong because, as it turned out, I was promoted within the year of returning. But my Dad unfortunately didn't help me to feel good about myself.'

It is difficult for spouses, family members or friends to know how best to help a stressed person through such a difficult time. Melissa C. Stoppler, a doctor who runs a health web site, is very aware that people closest to those undergoing chronic stress can also fall victim to that person's stress if they are not careful.[23] She suggests a number of ways for spouses and families to protect themselves from the stress being suffered by a loved one:

Protection from other people's stress

1. Don't take responsibility for another's stress.
2. Be honest with yourself and others. Discuss openly your concerns.
3. Accept someone else's tolerance for stress may be different from yours.
4. Keep a positive focus.
5. Refuse to feel guilty if you're not stressed too.
6. Suggest a vacation or activity you can do together.
7. Choose appropriate times for discussions with your spouse or friend on the subject of stress.
8. Don't take it personally if your concern or suggestions are not accepted. Back off and try again later.
9. Brighten their day by sending an unexpected plant or card.

The Effects on the Employer

Those signed off with work-related stress often ask themselves the same baffling question: why does their employer allow the situation to get to this stage? There would seem to be, at the very least, a financial benefit for a company in alleviating workers' stress. It is hugely expensive in terms of productivity for a member of staff to be unhappy in their work or at home on sick leave. If misery loves company, those suffering from stress can take solace in the knowledge that they are not alone – for their organization is suffering too!

For any member of staff who is unhappy at work – whether because of volume of work, bullying, finding themselves in the wrong job or dealing with a personal crisis – the employer must get to the root of the problem quickly and work out ways of solving it. The costs to a company, in terms of profit and productivity, are immense. First of all, the performance of an unhappy or stressed-out employee will be affected, with the result that he or she will be less productive. Mistakes may occur, absences for medical appointments and sick leave will ensure work is uncompleted, and the overall effect on the existing team may be demoralizing. Secondly, resentment towards both the person on sick leave and the employer may arise as those remaining are requested to cover the workload. This can in turn lead to employees feeling less loyal towards the company – or even to those remaining employees falling ill with stress, as Christine did when forced to cover for absent colleagues.

A stressed-out employee is, quite literally, a waste of time for a company. If an employee is being bullied, the time he or she takes away from doing a job – due to double-checking work, keeping records of events and minutes of meetings, and predicting possible areas of conflict before they happen – can be immense and protracted.

And not only time is lost. The costs of administering sick benefits, paying for an employee to see an occupational therapist, nurse and/or counsellor, will soon mount up. And if the employee eventually leaves, the employer loses out on the original recruitment costs, training investment, and the knowledge the employee brings. There is also the possibility of adverse publicity if the case goes to an Employment Tribunal; and depending on the final result, an employer might have to pay tribunal costs, enhancement to the employee's pension because of voluntary redundancy, or an exit package. To cap it all, the employer will then have to carry the costs once again for recruiting a replacement. And if the problem causing the stress in the first place has not been addressed, the employer and the new employee may discover to their mutual displeasure that history repeats itself. It is no wonder that many people suffering from work-related stress question their employer's sanity when the root causes of the work-related stress are not addressed.

... and on the State

It is not just the employer who loses out if an employee is suffering from work-related stress, because the cost to the State is also enormous. 32.9 million working days were lost in Britain between 2001-2002 due to job-related illnesses. The cost to the government of supporting regular trips to the G.P and subsidised medication is extremely high. If an employee takes time off on sick leave, it costs the government money to administer sick pay and provisions offered. According to recent government statistics, there are 2.4 million people in Britain claiming incapacity benefit, nearly one million of whom suffer from depression and anxiety and are too stressed to work.[24]

Furthermore, if an employee suffers so badly from work-related stress that he loses his job, then the State might have to provide incapacity or employment benefits. In some cases, a person might, on losing his income, likewise lose his house, leaving the government responsible for providing some sort of housing.

'Facts do not cease to exist because they are ignored,' as Aldous Huxley once wrote. It seems, therefore, that it is to no-one's benefit when an employee suffers from work-related stress. An employer and employee are dependent on each other, but both are personally responsible for their own decisions on how they respond to work situations. Taking responsibility for yourself means taking responsibility for how you fit into the working environment. And sometimes that situation, irrespective of how uncomfortable it feels, needs to be challenged or changed to ensure the well being of the work force.

3 WHAT ARE MY RIGHTS?

So … you are suffering from the symptoms of stress and have good reason to believe that your job is the culprit. Where do you stand from a legal point of view if you wish to claim sick leave or take your employer to court? Most people – unless it is part of their job to know details of employment law – are vague about their rights and responsibilities within the work place. It is only when something goes wrong that they begin to investigate their legal footing. However, prevention can be better than cure, and advance knowledge of responsibilities for both employers and employees might not only prevent a build-up of work-related stress, but create much better working relations between the managers and the managed.

You and the law

First of all, a quick caveat. All laws are fluid and subject to change. They are up-dated or repealed as, and when, society's (or the government's) attitudes change. However, everyone in the work place should have at least a basic knowledge of their legal rights – for example, how many hours they are required to work, how safe their working environment must be, and where they stand vis-à-vis discrimination. These laws will be discussed below and are valid at the time of publication. It is imperative, though, that you always check that the law discussed has not since been up-dated or amended by referring to a resource such as the TUC web site.[1]

How many hours must I work?

Working long hours, as we have seen, is a proven cause of work-related stress, and British workers put in the longest hours in Europe. The culture of working long hours is nothing new, of course. In 1907 the American labour campaigner Mary Van Kleeck wrote in her report, *Working Hours of Women in Factories,* that it was not uncommon for women, on top of running a household, to work a 78-hour week in factories in and around New York City. At the time the law in New York stated that women should work no longer than a 60-hour week, which Van Kleeck considered far too high. Things were somewhat better on the other side of the Atlantic. Thanks to the Factory Act of 1874, British workers toiled in factories for only ten hours a day. And some British employers were remarkably progressive. In 1893 the Salford Iron Works of Mather and Platt in Manchester established the 8-hour day. Eleven years later, in 1904, the firm reported: 'Our experience since the first year in which it (the eight hour system) was tried has fully borne out the conclusions then arrived at, and we are fully satisfied that as regards the comparison between 8 and 9 hours per day, the balance of advantage is in favour of the shorter period'.[2] The iron works was more productive, in other words, when the employees worked shorter hours.

American employers in New York were not so forward-thinking. Van Kleeck did not manage to reduce the long working hours for women to an 8-hour day, but her comments supporting her case are as valid today as they were back in 1907: 'To the community a worn-out worker is an economic loss. So is the man who, by wearing out the community's workers, underbids his competitors and lowers the whole standard of trade conditions'.

Van Kleeck's argument is especially relevant today, and UK business groups would do well to heed her words. Under the Working Time Directive, all EU member states must ensure that employees do not work longer than an average of 48 hours a week. However, in 1993 the British government under John Major secured the right for UK businesses to broker volunteer deals with employees, allowing them to work more than 48 hours a week if they so wished. This is commonly known as the 'opt-out'.

However, the days of this opt-out could be numbered since in February 2004 MEPs in Brussels voted in support of the European Commission's proposals to enforce the 48-hour limit in *all* EU countries. The Confederation of British Industry (CBI) responded by saying this move would be a 'serious blow' to employees' rights to govern their time. Still, it seems that many employees do not actually have the right to govern their time in the work place as the CBI argues, since according to a TUC poll in 2003, one in three of those who signed an opt-out agreement claim they were given no choice in the matter. Furthermore, two out of three who regularly work more than 48 hours a week say they have not been asked to opt-out! So the idea of consensual opting-out of the 48-hours-a-week minimum is a bit of a fairy tale.

It is disheartening to think that, a century after both the Salford Iron Works and Mary Van Kleeck recognised the overall benefits of shorter working days, British business leaders are pushing for increased hours at the office in the name of 'labour flexibility' – and this at a time when 32.9 million working days are being lost every year due to work-related illnesses.[3]

So let's look closely at the UK law on working hours. And remember: if you think you are being exploited, you can ultimately challenge your employer in an Employment Tribunal:

- You cannot be forced to work more than 48 hours a week.
- You can agree with your employer to work more than 48 hours a week
  – an 'opt-out' – but this must be in writing and you must sign it.

- There is no opt-out for workers aged between 16 and 17 years old.
- Workers can cancel the opt-out agreement whenever they want, although they must give their employer at least seven days' warning.
- The average working time is normally calculated over 17 weeks, but this can be longer in certain situations (26 weeks) and extended (up to 52 weeks).
- Working time includes travelling where it is part of the job, working lunches, and job-related training. Working time does not include travelling between home and work.
- You are entitled to:
  - four weeks' paid holiday a year
  - a break when the working day is more than six hours
  - a rest period of 11 hours every working day
  - a rest period of 24 hours once every seven days
  - a maximum average of eight hours night work in every 24
  - a free health assessment for night workers.

I want to be flexible

Parenthood is not, it seems, an altogether attractive proposition for many people in the twenty-first century. One in five women in western Europe is childless, and the UK census of 2001 shows that, for the first time in England and Wales, there are more people over the age of 60 (20.9 per cent of the population) than children (20.2 per cent). Just over half the adult population (aged 16 and over) of England and Wales remains single, whilst separated or divorced people make up 10.6 per cent.[4] There is no indication that this trend will change, which is a worrying development for a government already facing an aging population and a shrinking workforce.

What is causing this drop in the birth rate? Critics of this decline in the traditional family blame a number of factors: ease of divorce, an increase in single parents, and the financial pressures on mothers of young children to enter the workforce. Added to these are other factors, such as inflexible work patterns for parents, too little time off for maternity or paternity leave, and the culture of long working hours, all of which are woefully incompatible with family life. As most parents can attest, a hectic home life – caring for children or elderly parents, for example – can lead to stress at the office. And, indeed, a recent study emphasises that 'family matters reduce the amount of sleep or time that the respondent can relax, and that these factors are reflected in higher work stress'.[5]

Armed with evidence that the family is breaking down and that women in the UK are having fewer children, the government has worked hard to introduce new laws to encourage parents not only to start having children again, but to be able to balance work with their home lives to enable more time for the family. All of which is good news, given the fact that, as we saw in Chapter One, a stressful personal life often carries over into the work place, affecting both the company's productivity and the worker's health.

The British Prime Minister, Tony Blair, grew so concerned about the effects of long hours in the office on the health of the British population that in March 2000 he launched the 'Work-Life Balance' campaign. The campaign was aimed at convincing employers of the enormous benefits of balancing employees' work and personal lives. A relaxed and happy staff, it was reasoned, can only work to the benefit of a company, with fewer workers taking sick leave or unexplained absences. Intriguingly, the Founder and President of the Work-Life Balance Trust is Shirley Conran, famous for her 1970 international best-seller *Superwoman,* which advised women how to cut down on the household chores in order to concentrate on their careers: 'Life is too short to stuff a mushroom' was her rallying cry. Ironically, Conran was actually suffering from ME/Chronic Fatigue Syndrome – an illness that has afflicted her for over 30 years – and wrote the book to help sufferers like herself. The publishers hid Conran's illness from the public, promoting the book as required reading for the woman who can do anything. They also deleted from the book a chapter on stress, arguing that her readers would not know what it was. Over thirty years later, readers have certainly learned the meaning of the term!

In January 2003, Patricia Hewitt, Secretary of State for Trade and Industry, speaking at a conference in London, reiterated the government's concern about the huge costs the UK incurs because of long working hours. One way of tackling the problem of overwork, according to Hewitt, is instituting flexible working. Her argument is supported by the *Bristol Stress and Health at Work Study,* which found that a significant correlation exists between levels of stress and powers of decision-making. Respondents in the high stress groups had little autonomy in deciding when to take a break and when to take holidays. Those in the low stress groups, conversely, reported much greater flexibility in their working conditions.[6]

So what do we mean by flexible working? It can include: (a) teleworking – working at home or off-site, up to but not more than a few days a week; (b) remote working – working almost exclusively off-site as the employee does not have an office facility at any company site; (c) part-time working – working less than the standard number of hours; (d) job sharing – two people sharing the responsibilities of one position; (e) a compressed working week – working the same number of hours, but in fewer days; and (f) flexitime – employees adjusting the time that they start and finish their shifts.

Large companies that have successfully introduced flexible working – Merck Pharmaceuticals (US and Spain), Peugeot (France), Unilever (UK) – have all consulted their employees about the type of flexibility they would prefer. All recognise that flexible working measures benefit their businesses in terms of both productivity and loyalty.[7]

Several months after Hewitt's speech, in April 2003, the government introduced new legislation to help working parents juggle their lives and careers. This legislation included the right to request flexible working, parental leave, maternity leave (updated), paternity leave (updated), adoption leave (updated) and family emergency leave. The law can be summarized point-by-point:

- *The right to request flexible working:* Parents of children under the age of six or of disabled children under the age of 18 will have the right to apply to work flexibly providing they have worked the qualifying length of service – 26 weeks. Employers will have a statutory duty to consider their applications and a procedure is in place for employers to follow, but the employee does not have an automatic right to work flexibly if an employer cannot accommodate the changes.

- *Parental leave:* Each parent (including adoptive parents), providing they have worked for their employer for one year, can take up to 13 weeks (unpaid) leave to care for a child under the age of five years old. For adoptive parents it must be taken within five years from the date of placement. Parents of disabled children are entitled to 18 weeks (unpaid) leave up until the child's 18th birthday. This leave must be taken in blocks of at least a week, and no more than four weeks can be taken in any single year. You must give 21 days notice and your employer can make you postpone it for up to six months.

- *Maternity leave:* The length of 'ordinary maternity leave' (paid leave) is 26 weeks and can be extended for a further 26 weeks (unpaid) if you have completed 26 weeks' continuous service by the beginning of the 14th week before the expected week of childbirth (EWC). The earliest date you can commence your maternity leave is the beginning of the 11th EWC.

- *Paternity leave:* If you have or expect to have responsibility for the child's upbringing, if you are the biological father or the mother's husband or partner and you have worked continuously for your employer for 26 weeks, then you are eligible to take paternity leave (paid) for up to two weeks. It can be taken in one or two week blocks but not in single days and within 56 days of the EWC.

- *Adoptive parent leave:* Individuals or one member of a couple who adopt are eligible for paid adoptive parent leave. The other partner of a couple can claim paid paternity leave. Adopters are entitled to 26 weeks 'ordinary adoption leave' which can be extended for up to 26 weeks of additional adoption leave (unpaid).

- *Family emergency leave:* All employees are also entitled to take a reasonable amount of (unpaid) time off work to deal with an emergency or unexpected situation involving a dependent whether a minor or elderly relative.

Looking after my health and safety

Some jobs, as we have seen, can be more stressful than others. But nobody will be surprised to learn that a dangerous or unhealthy job is also usually a stressful one. Workers whose jobs expose them to noxious fumes, dusts and other potentially harmful substances have, a recent study has found, high levels of stress, as do those exposed to loud or constant noises in the work place.[8] Anyone in these sorts of employment, therefore, must be on intimate terms with current health and safety legislation if they are to ensure that their stress levels – and their health – are not prejudiced. Forewarned, as always, is forearmed.

The basis of British health and safety law stems from the *Health and Safety at Work* Act 1974, while *The Management of Health and Safety at Work regulations 1999* clarifies what employers are required to do to ensure your health, safety and welfare at work.

Under health and safety law your employer must ensure:

- You are not injured or made ill at work.
- You are given the information, instruction, training and supervision necessary for your health and safety.
- You are consulted on any change that may substantially affect your health and safety at work.
- Your work place has an accident book in which work-related injuries are recorded.
- A risk assessment is carried out in your work place and if there are five or more employees this should be recorded.

As an employee, you also have legal duties:

- You must work safely and co-operate with your employer following safety guidelines.

Remember that you have a right to refuse to do something dangerous. If your employer disciplines you, you are entitled to compensation. If you think that your employer is not carrying out their legal duties or is exposing you to risks, you must in the first instance point this out to them. There are all sorts of reasons why employers might deny your rights. Sometimes they are simply ignorant of the law and their responsibilities, and once challenged, will put the situation right. Whatever their reasons, however, if they do not respond to your concerns you can contact either your union rep, your health and safety adviser or, failing that, the Health and Safety Executive's

Info-line (0521 545500). *Remember that if you do not first discuss the problem with your manager you will not have a case legally.*

Discrimination

Work-related stress can be caused by discrimination in any form, and laws have been passed to try to stop discrimination against employees on any grounds other than their ability to do the job. It is, therefore, illegal to discriminate against anyone on grounds of race, colour, nationality, ethnic origins, religion, philosophical belief, gender, marital status, pregnancy, actual or perceived sexual orientation, disability, or their desire for part-time work; and in 2006 it will be illegal to discriminate on the grounds of age. For specific help and advice contact the Equal Opportunities Commission[9], the Commission for Racial Equality,[10] the Disability Rights Commission,[11] the Employers' Forum on Disability,[12] and Acas (Advisory, Conciliation and Arbitration Scheme).[13]

However, at present it is not possible to make a direct complaint to an employment tribunal about bullying, so if your situation does not fit into any of the above categories – for example, you are a woman being bullied by a manager for unspecified reasons – you are still protected under sections 44 and 100 of the *Employment Rights Act 1996*, which states that employees have the right:

- not to be disadvantaged
- to raise health and safety concerns with the employer (e.g. complaining about a workplace bully)
- to take 'protective action', or even to leave work, in the circumstances of 'serious imminent danger'.[14]

What this means is that your employer must ensure that the work place is a safe environment for all employees. If a worker is being bullied and harassed so much that they feel their only option is to leave, they can claim 'constructive dismissal'. Also, as discussed earlier, under the *Health and Safety at Work Act 1974* employers are responsible for the health, safety and welfare at work of *all* employees, so it might be proved that an employer is in breach of contract for failing to protect an employee's health and safety at work. Always take advice from your union rep or from an independent solicitor before taking action if you are thinking of claiming 'constructive dismissal'. Make sure that you have a strong case before being forced into this last resort.

What happens if I am laid off?

As we have seen from the previous chapter, being on the receiving end of a P45 can be a cause of work-related stress. It is useful to know, therefore, where you stand legally and what an employer can and cannot do when laying off workers. First of all, you must be clear whether you are classified as an 'employee' or 'worker/self-employed'. An employee is usually given a contract of employment, which may be for a specific period of time. Alternatively, you are classified as a worker if you carry out a particular task in return for a fee – a 'contract for services'. Your employment rights under either contract are enforceable by law.

You need to check your contract of employment as sometimes your employment rights kick in or improve after a stated period of time. However, for redundancy to be legal it must adhere to the following principles:

- You are only redundant if your job ends and no-one else is hired to do the same job.
- Employers may select people for redundancy but they cannot discriminate on the grounds of sex, race or disability.
- If there are more than 20 redundancies in one year, then your employer must consult the workforce. If there is no union, then special reps should be elected who can negotiate on your behalf.

You are entitled to redundancy pay if you have worked for your employer for longer than two years. When giving staff redundancy pay, many employers are more generous than the legal requirement, but the amount will depend on your salary, age and length of service. The minimum is as follows:

- aged 18-21 – half a week's pay for each year of service
- aged 22-40 – one week's pay for each year of service
- aged 40-65 – one and a half week's pay for each year of service
- Weekly pay of more than £240 is not counted and no more than 20 years service can be taken into account.

If your employer does not follow the law as laid out above, you are entitled to challenge them in an Employment Tribunal. Details of tribunals are covered later in this chapter. However, if you are in a union you can ask your rep for advice or contact your local Citizen's Advice Bureau, a local law centre, or ACAS (Advisory, Conciliation, Arbitration Scheme) – a government funded service for employees and employers. Contacts are at the back of the book.

Taking sick leave

It is not necessary to handle hazardous materials or breathe noxious fumes in order to be made ill by your job. As we saw in the previous chapter, the effects of prolonged stress, so prevalent in modern life, can make some people so ill they need to take sick leave to heal.

The decision to take sick leave is not always a simple or straightforward one. For some employees, the very thought of taking time off sick can add to their existing stress levels, as they fear this 'truancy' might lead to dismissal. And in some cases this does indeed occur because, let's face it, your employer loses money every day you are away from work. An employer has two options if you go off on long-term sick leave: either to assist in getting you back to work as soon as possible by introducing measures that will counteract the cause of your stress; or to sack you and find a replacement. The latter can be done without fear of litigation only if the employer has followed set dismissal procedures and can prove that your absence threatens the business – and in a small business, with a small workforce, this claim would not be unrealistic. If, however, the employer *cannot* prove that your absence threatens the survival of the business, then you can claim unfair dismissal and take your employer to an industrial tribunal.

So how much time can you reasonably take off on sick leave and how much can you expect to be paid during this period? Under the *Statutory Sick Pay Act 1994, all employees,* full-time or part-time, who are unable to work because of sickness, and who earn enough to qualify, are eligible for statutory sick pay (SSP), of which an employer can claim part back from the government. SSP is payable for up to 28 weeks in any one year apart from the first three days of an illness, and these unpaid days are known as 'waiting days'. The standard rate for SSP in 2004 is £64.35 per week. If you are still unable to work after 28 weeks, you must claim Incapacity Benefit from Social Security.

An employee may 'self-certify'[15] his illness for the first seven days, and Business Link, an advice organisation for employers, advises that employees should be asked to be specific on their certificate about why they are off sick. They also advise that sickness should be monitored and all employees should be interviewed on their return to check that the system is not abused. Under the rules of SSP, employees are required to produce a doctor's certificate after seven days on sick leave – and this includes weekends and public holidays. However, it is wise to check your employment contract as many employers pay what is known as 'contractual sick pay', which usually means normal wages from the first day of absence, rather than making the first three days unpaid, and regular pay for the time you are off on sick leave. As long as the minimum SSP rates are paid and payment periods are adhered to, the employer can specify how much is paid and for how long. This must, however, be made clear in your contract of employment.

It should be noted that, in order to curb those suspected of feigning illness, there is presently a trend for employers to withhold sickness pay for three 'waiting days'. The supermarket chains Asda and Tesco, who have experimented with this approach, claim that sickness rates – especially those falling on a Monday or Friday – have been dramatically reduced. Fair enough treatment, perhaps, for malingerers hoping for a day off work at their employer's expense. However, withholding pay for three days from those genuinely suffering from work-related stress will not necessarily coerce them back into the work place. So if you find yourself in this situation, talk it through with your doctor. A medical professional will not be able to offer you any financial compensation for those three days without pay, but he or she will be able to assess the severity of your symptoms. A good employer will not abandon you if you are off on long-term sick leave so long as you have your doctor's backing. It is very costly for them to re-advertise your job and retrain someone else. Business Link therefore advises employers to arrange progress reports and home visits and to reassure the employee there is a job to come back to. An employer might suggest you return on a part-time basis for a short period or be given lighter duties for a while to ease you back into work. However, as long as the consequences of wilful absenteeism are spelt out in the disciplinary procedures, an employer can withhold SSP if they reasonable suspect an employee is not really ill. If after four or more absences in a year an employer suspects his employee is not genuinely ill he can seek an 'adjudication' from the Inland Revenue Medical Services. Refusal to allow the Inland Revenue Medical Service to become involved may be grounds for employee's SSP to be stopped.

Ultimately, you can be dismissed for reasons of sickness if your employer can show that he has considered all the alternatives – easing you back into work, tackling the cause of your stress – and meanwhile consulted you in the process. In a large firm, dismissal won't usually occur until the full 28-week SSP period is up, but in a small firm, where a gap in the staff could threaten business, it might be sooner.

However daunting some of these rules and regulations might seem, taking time off for work-related stress is the only alternative for many people. The negative effects of stress can be extremely serious to your long-term health, so a visit to your doctor is imperative. Doctors are professionals with a wealth of experience, and most are quite capable of distinguishing between a malingerer and someone who is genuinely ill. If you require time out of work to heal, then your doctor will certainly advise it!

What happens if I am disciplined?

Providing an employer has attempted to take measures to reduce the cause of your stress in the work place, and follows the correct disciplinary process, you can be fired if your employer proves that due to sickness you are no longer 'capable' of doing your job. This is not much peace of mind if you are too ill to work, but many employers will bend over backwards to help you to return to work, and dismissal is often only a last resort.

From October 2004, all firms are obliged to have minimum statutory procedures in place for dealing with disputes, grievances and dismissals. The procedures are included in the Employment Act 2002 (Dispute Resolution Regulations) and are an attempt to reduce the number of cases that go to Employment Tribunals. Previously, firms with fewer than 20 employees had been exempt from providing staff with information on disciplinary and grievance procedures but now they too must comply. The process therefore is as follows:

Dismissal and Disciplinary Procedure (DPP)

Step 1 – The employer writes to the employee giving details of their concerns. A meeting is arranged to discuss it.

Step 2 – A meeting takes place prior to any disciplinary action being taken.

Step 3 – The employer informs the employee of their decision. If the employee wants to appeal, the employer must hold a further meeting. After this hearing the employer must inform the employee of their decision.

- There is a modified approach for employees that have been dismissed for misconduct.

The Standard Grievance Procedure (SGP)

Step 1 – The employee must write to the employer about the grievance.

Step 2 – A meeting is arranged by the employer to discuss the grievance. The employer decides the outcome.

Step 3 – The employee can appeal against the employer's decision. The employer must organise an appeal hearing. The employer informs the employee of their decision.

- There is a modified approach for employees that have already left the company.

It is important for both the employer and employee to follow the statutory procedures in a case for dismissal. An employer who fails to adhere to these procedures will be guilty of 'unfair dismissal', while the employee who has not, in the first instance, written to his employer outlining his grievance will find that his complaint will not be upheld.

If you are still not happy with the outcome of your dismissal you have two options:

providing both parties are in agreement, you can agree to participate in the Acas (Advisory, Conciliation and Arbitration Services) Arbitration Scheme or, if you are sure of your legal position, you can take your case to an Employment Tribunal. In this case you do not need the backing of your employer.

Employment Tribunals: how useful are they?

If, as discussed above, you are unhappy with the results of the DPP, the SGP or any other aspect of your employment relations, you can take your case to an Employment Tribunal. Tribunal hearings usually take place before a legally qualified chairman (nominated by Acas) and two lay members. Both the employer and employee's representatives nominate these lay members, who could be union reps or personnel officers. The aim is for the process to be impartial. Decisions are made by the majority vote, but in most cases agreements are unanimous. The Acas Code of Practice is the yardstick for unfair dismissal cases, but statute law is adhered to. Employment tribunals have their own rules, however, and the burden of proof is lighter than in the courts. For example, hearsay evidence can be admitted and you do not have to prove anything 'beyond a reasonable doubt'.

Employment Tribunals are not always satisfactory because they can take a long time and are potentially very costly. From October 2004 Employment Tribunals have involved the introduction of mandatory tribunal forms, and the exchange of documents has been speeded up in an attempt to encourage early dispute resolution. The government has introduced these measures because statistics show that 44% of people leave their jobs through either resignations or dismissals – a huge expense to both employers and employees.[16] However, these new measures notwithstanding, you need to think carefully whether you want to put yourself through the months of increased stress and tension – especially as, in some cases, you might be able to negotiate a agreed settlement without going to court.

The Acas Arbitration Scheme

Provided both parties agree, there is an alternative procedure to Employment Tribunals. This is the Acas Arbitration Scheme that operates in England and Wales (and in Scotland since October 2004). It is an informal, non-confrontational procedure overseen by an impartial adviser from Acas employers' advice organisation. The beauty of this approach is, first of all, that it is not open to the public, and second, that it is quick compared to a Tribunal, usually being completed within an afternoon. The venue is often a local hotel. Awards, if granted, use the same guidelines as a Tribunal. The Arbitration Scheme cannot be used in cases of sexual discrimination or non-payment of wages, but its remit covers unfair dismissal and flexible working conditions.[17]

Before you go to an Employment Tribunal ...

- Be aware that each side generally pays its own legal costs regardless of who wins the case. Also, if you have already been warned at a pre-hearing review that your claim has no reasonable prospect of success, you might be asked to contribute to the other side's legal costs.

- An unfair dismissal case might cost £1,500 to £2,000 to defend. A discrimination case could cost £15,000. An applicant cannot obtain legal aid, except to help in preparing a claim. In some cases your union might fight your corner and pay the fees.

- Check whether your case is not technically flawed – in unfair dismissal cases you must be employed for a full year and make a claim within three months of the termination date. Note that if your employer discovers the claim is invalid on technical grounds, they can write to the tribunal and ask for a preliminary hearing to have the claim thrown out. If a pre-hearing review is set, the weaker case may be ordered to pay a deposit of up to £500 before continuing with the claim.

- Investigate whether a settlement can be agreed before going to a Tribunal. Awards are unpredictable, especially in discrimination cases, and an employer may think a settlement is a better option than experiencing the disruption and damage to the business in terms of morale and management time. Also, it means you won't have to relive the dreadful experience as you prepare your case for the Tribunal.

If, after having weighed up the options, you are determined to go ahead with a Tribunal, the process is as follows:

- The applicant submits a form (IT1) to a regional tribunal office. The complaint is made and states whether reinstatement or compensation is required. The employer is sent a copy and must respond on another form (IT3) within 21 days. The employer can request longer than 21 days to respond if the case is complicated.

- The date for the hearing will be set, and the employer is sometimes only given a couple of weeks' notice. They must respond within 14 days. An impartial conciliator from Acas assigned to the case will try to work out ways the two sides can come to an agreement.

- All documents usually are exchanged before the hearing – witness statements and other relevant papers. You will need at least six photocopies of each paper.

- The hearing is public and open to the press. In the case of unfair dismissal, the employer usually goes first; in a discrimination case it is the applicant who begins.

- Both sides can have witnesses who, if called by either side, are compelled to attend the hearing to submit to questioning.

- A decision is usually announced at the end of the case or within a few days, and both sides receive the adjudication in writing. If either side does not like the tribunal's decision, they can ask for it to be reviewed as long as they do so within 14 days of the original decision.

- You can take the case to an Employment Appeal Tribunal if you do so within six weeks of the original adjudication, but most decisions are made on a point of law and few appeals are successful.

The average award as a result of a Tribunal is only £3,000, so you should think carefully before you embark on this course of action as most likely you will have to pay your costs, which may well exceed this amount. Financial awards can be separated into 'unfair dismissal', 'breach of contract' and 'discrimination', and the amounts vary depending on the case.

Unfair dismissal is made up of two elements: A basic award which, as of February 2004, is capped at £8,100 and takes into account age and service; and a compensatory award based on the loss of past and future earnings and how unfair the dismissal was. These awards, from February 2004, are capped at £55,000.

Breach of contract awards are capped at £25,000.

Discrimination awards are unlimited. They take into account loss of earnings and injury to feelings.

However, it is risky to rely on receiving a large financial settlement from a Tribunal, as most cases are never completely clear-cut. So agreeing a settlement before reaching a Tribunal may be in your better interest. A settlement may include a cash sum and a reference with agreed wording. A confidentiality clause may also be part of the deal, something you cannot expect from a Tribunal no matter who wins.

There are two ways in which a settlement can be reached. Acas can draw up a legally binding agreement known as a COT3 settlement, or a 'compromise agreement' is composed. These were introduced so that unscrupulous employers could not make their employees 'sign away' their employment rights unless specific processes were in place. If these rules are not adhered to, both types of agreements are null and void.

The COT3 is a standard form the Acas conciliation officer uses to formally record the settlement. Providing an employee receives independent legal advice he can waive his statutory employment rights in return for an agreed settlement. These agreements are legally binding and the employer usually pays the employee's legal costs of up to £330.[18]

Compromise agreements, on the other hand were introduced when Acas became increasingly reluctant to involve itself in cases where a formal complaint to a tribunal had not been presented. There is no need for an Acas conciliation officer to be involved in drawing up a compromise agreement, but the following rules must be adhered to:

- The agreement must be in writing and relate specifically to the complaint in question.
- The employee must have independent advice from a qualified lawyer, a trade union official appropriately qualified and authorised by the union, or an advice centre worker who is appropriately certified and authorised.
- The agreement must identify this independent adviser.
- There must be an insurance policy in force covering the independent adviser at time of giving advice.
- The advice given to the employee must cover the 'terms and effect' of the proposed agreement.
- The agreement must cover in writing all that has been agreed.

Unions: how useful are they?

Workers' rights in Britain have come a long way since George Loveless and the Tolpuddle Martyrs were deported to Tasmania in 1834 for setting up the Friendly Society of Agricultural Labourers. Union membership in 2002 was recorded at 7.3 million, and in 2004 there were 230,000 union reps in the work place. However, union membership has virtually halved since it was at its peak in 1979, when there were 13.5 million members and 500,000 union reps. Does this mean that unions are losing their power? And how helpful can they be in taking up your cause?

To answer this question it is useful to take a brief look at the history of the union in twentieth-century Britain in order to understand how the present laws that protect you have arisen, why they have not gone further to protect your rights in the work place, and why some critics argue that the employer still has the upper hand.

A combination of circumstances led to the unions' decline, starting with the 'Social Contract' they agreed with the Labour government of James Callaghan in the mid-1970s, in which pay increases were kept down in order to protect the 'national interest' by damping down inflation. Low-paid workers couldn't keep up with galloping inflation – which their stunted pay packets had done nothing to control – and so went on strike, culminating in the 'Winter of Discontent' of 1978-79. As a consequence of the inconveniences caused by the strikes, large numbers of voters opted for a change of government, ensuring that the Tories under Margaret Thatcher won the May 1979 election. Mass unemployment and industrial closures in the 1980s ignited more strikes – steel in 1981, miners in 1984, printers in 1985, ferry workers in 1988. However, the Conservative government, backed by employers, brought in a series of anti-union laws to curb resistance. These laws[19] were designed to stop unions from implementing the principle of solidarity – i.e., everyone out on strike even if the membership didn't unanimously agree to down tools – and secondary action if striking failed to achieve the outcome desired. Unions now face fines for unlawful action.[20] The Labour government of Tony Blair, elected in 1997 and re-elected four years later, has not repealed these laws.

Modern-day unions have changed their tactics, moving away from collective action against employers and towards campaigning for the creation and implementation of legal mechanisms to protect the worker. Though they might not have the protection from a union individuals now have the legal means to challenge employers if they are being abused in the work place. The various laws the Labour government has recently introduced or updated – minimum wage; maternity, paternity and adoption leave and pay; redundancy notice and pay; arbitration and employment tribunal rules; the disciplinary and grievance process; discrimination and health and safety legislation – mark a successful attempt to remove the necessity of collective action by having clear legal guidelines for both employers and employees to follow.

Many of these new rights have been won by union campaigning, but in the best work places unions and employers work together, and the emphasis is on negotiation rather than confrontation. As the TUC explains, British Unions 'have put behind them outdated ideas of confrontation and now aim to work together with employers in partnership.'[21] Likewise, employers have increasingly begun to recognise that if their morale and commitment can be improved, staff are more likely to be committed to their work and more ready to embrace the changes needed to compete in a modern world – something that the managers of the Salford Iron Works of Mather and Platt discovered over a hundred years ago when they reduced their working days from the statutory ten hours to eight.

So, how useful is it, these days, to be a member of a union? Although these new employment laws are a long stride in the right direction, there is no doubt that having union backing puts you in a stronger bargaining position for enforcing your statutory rights. Being a member of a union helps in two particular ways: First of all, under the 1999 *Employment Relations Act* an employee is permitted to bring a companion, who may be a trade union official, to any disciplinary or grievance hearing – something that can be of great advantage. Secondly, if your case goes to an Employment Tribunal, you might not be out of pocket as often a union will pay your legal fees. Financing legal representation yourself might be not only expensive but your lawyer may be less informed than a union rep about the 'ins and outs' of your work place.

Not everyone, it should be noted, has the option of union representation. The 1999 *Employment Relations Act* states that any work place with more than 21 employees has the right to union representation if so requested. However, 21.8% of the UK workforce are in establishments with less than 19 staff and therefore do not have that right. They do, however, have the benefit of all of the protective measures spelled out in this chapter.

The Data Protection Act: what does it mean?

In Chapter Four we will explore the role professionals such as doctors, counsellors and occupational nurses have in helping you overcome work-related stress. Some people, however, are hesitant to make use of these invaluable resources. One reservation many employees have about consulting such experts is the fear of what might be done with their confidential information. For example, what would happen to your career within the company if details of your diagnosis of depression, recorded by the occupational nurse, were leaked to your manager and fellow employees?

Theoretically, you should have nothing to fear as the law on confidentiality states very clearly how any such information about you can and cannot be used. If this trust is abused you can sue through a civil court and the offender can be struck off their professional or medical register. Article 8 of the European Convention of Human Rights, now incorporated into the *Human Rights Acts* of 1998, and the *Data Protection Act* of 1998, both clearly state that your privacy is guaranteed, and that all sensitive information, whether computerised or manually written, is stored and distributed, where appropriate, only in the strictest of confidence.[22] The sole exceptions are if the health-care professional concerned thinks that you are either a danger to yourself or others, or a terrorist. Personal details that support these assumptions can be divulged where necessary.[23]

The *Data Protection Act* of 1998 states people have a right to know when information about them is collected for use and the purpose for gathering it must be stated. This means that you have a right of access to personal data and can have inaccuracies corrected, removed or destroyed. It is the responsibility of the professional that collects such information to ensure any such records are kept confidential and locked up. The *Computer Misuse* Act 1990 preceded the *Data Protection Act* and came into force to secure computer programs and data against unauthorised access or alteration. It is therefore a criminal offence if those users go beyond what is permitted and disclose information. But it is the doctor, counsellor, occupational nurse or data-processor, and not the employer, who is accountable for the information, and they are the ones who could be sued. Unless you give your consent, this information cannot be shared with anyone else. This should reassure you that any information you decide to share with a doctor, counsellor or occupational nurse will remain confidential. Not even your employer has a right to know unless you give your consent!

References: where do I stand?

If you have lost your job or taken extended sick leave due to work-related stress, where do you stand regarding to a reference from your employer? Is an employer legally obliged to give you a reference? If you have left under a cloud, what exactly is your employer allowed to write about your situation, and are you entitled to see the reference? More importantly, what can you do if you think your reference has been unfair and has therefore affected your chances of finding employment elsewhere?

Unfortunately - or maybe fortunately, depending on your point of view - an employer is not obliged to provide you with a reference. If one is given, as long as the employer believes it to be correct and without malice, it is protected by what is known in the legal field as 'qualified privilege'. This means that the information between the two parties - you and your employer - is not subject to legal scrutiny. However, if information that you know to be untrue is provided in the reference, or if the statement falls into the hands of a third person who does not have a valid interest in the matter, then 'qualified privilege' does not protect the employer. Therefore, it is sensible for a referee to take care when writing a reference, as he will be held negligent if he fails to do so and if the employee suffers as a consequence.

As explained in the previous section on the Data Protection Act, you are allowed access to information held on you by an organisation. However, employment references are excluded from this right under section 7 of the Act due to the fact that a reference is sent in confidence to a named person, usually in another company. If you are concerned about the content, you can apply to your new or potential employer – not to your old one – for a copy of the reference.

There are exceptions under section 7 which give you access to a reference and they are as follows:

- References given by a third party (e.g. a former employer) that are held in an employee's current personnel file. In most cases an employer would have to acquire the former employer's consent first before disclosure. If the former employer refuses to give his consent, the recipient of the reference must decide whether the benefit of disclosure outweighs the duty of confidentiality.

- The *Access to Medical Reports Act 1988* gives patients the right of access to reports prepared for insurance or employment purposes. This is important if you have had time off for work-related stress and your employer gives this as the reason for your absence. However, if your employer mentions that you have had a certain number of weeks off on sick leave and does not mention the reason why, your employer in this situation does not have to show you their reference first because he has not divulged confidential information without your consent. However, you might be asked directly by your new employer the reasons for your absence.

- If the reference is compiled by a Credit Reference Agency for a loan and you are refused on the basis of their reference, you have the right, under the *Consumer Credit Act 1974*, to ask the Credit Reference Agency to see a copy of the reference. You can correct any inconsistencies, but it remains up to the loan company whether they accept you for a loan.

What can you do if, after getting access to a reference, you believe it to be unfair and harmful to your chances of finding further employment? Well, it will depend on what is wrong with it.

- **Defamation** – This is actually quite difficult to prove in court but means that your reference gives a false impression that amounts to a character slur, and is given with malicious intent.

- **Injurious falsehood** – Similar to defamation, but malice – which need not simply be a slur on your character - must be shown.

- **Negligent mis-statement** – This is more likely to succeed in Court and arose from the case (Spring v Guardian Assurance plc & ors 1994 ICR 596)[24] where the Lords ruled that an employer who gives a reference is under a duty to take reasonable care in the preparation of that reference and would be liable to the employee in negligence if the reference was inaccurate and the employee suffered loss as a result.

In this latter case, ruled on by the Law Lords, S was dismissed from his job as an insurance sales manager. He applied for a similar position with another insurance company but was not offered the job on receipt of his reference from his current employer. The reference stated that S was dishonest and had tried to sell a client an unsuitable insurance policy in order to maximise his own commission. This reference was described as the 'kiss of death' for S's chances of future employment in this field. The Lords ruled that S was not acting dishonestly and that his employer also wrote the reference honestly, believing in the statements made. The Court ruled that the employer and his company owed a duty of care to the employee in the making of the reference and that this duty was breached. As a result of this case, employers must now take 'reasonable care and skill' to ensure that the accuracy of the facts written or communicated in a reference does not cause a potential employer to form an adverse opinion on the employee.[25] Employers must also ensure that the information provided is not misleading.[26]

Employers can now find themselves in a difficult situation when writing references, as on the one hand they must ensure that the picture painted will not blight the future prospects of an employee, yet they must ensure, on the other hand, that nothing is omitted from the reference that might over exaggerate the employee's abilities. Someone who recruited an employee on the basis of a good reference that then turns out to be inaccurate may suffer a loss as a result – in terms of recruitment expenses, ability for the job to be done – and can then take legal action against the referee. To shield themselves against potential litigation, employers can now agree to write a reference only if the employee accepts that there will be a disclaimer of liability to him or her and to the recipient of the reference. This is feasible due to a 'compromise agreement' that is negotiated on termination, but it must satisfy the requirement of 'reasonableness' under Section 2 of the *Unfair Contract Terms Act 1977*,[27] otherwise it too will not hold up in court. There is not a strict definition of the term 'reasonableness', but it usually is assessed with reference to what the parties could be expected to know when the contract was formed.[28]

So if your employers agree to give you a reference, what can they safely write about you? 'Get the facts, or the facts will get you,' as the proverb says. 'And when you get them, get them right, or they will get you wrong.'[29] A standard reference can include:

- Length of service and position held
- Competence on the job
- Honesty
- Time-keeping
- Lengthy period of absences
- Any remarks of a more personal nature can be made as long that they are based on accurate facts

Regarding competence on the job, if reference is made to poor performance, this must have been previously discussed with the employee, as shown in the case of TSB Bank plc v. Harris. H applied for a job at the Prudential whilst working at TSB but failed to get the job because of her reference. The reference stated that 17 complaints had been made against H, four of which were upheld and eight were outstanding. H had only been told about two of the complaints, the remaining 15 had never been discussed with her.

As an employer is not *obliged* to write you a reference, provisions for one might be something to include in negotiations with your employer if you are going to try for an exit package. An employer will often agree to write the minimum facts about job title and length of service. If, on the other hand, your employer refuses to write a reference, well … the end of the world is not nigh! Contact previous employers for references and supply them instead to your prospective employers. If questioned by a potential employer, do not hesitate to be honest, especially if you feel you are not in the wrong. However, be brief and do not go into petty details about your problems with your previous employer! Explain that you tried to negotiate changes to the cause of your work-related stress but were unsuccessful. If a potential employer refuses to employ you because of such a past history, ask yourself if you honestly wish to work for someone that might be similar in attitude to your previous employer? There are plenty of employers willing to work in ways that suit you.

It is important to remember that a reference does not 'make the man', and a successful application has more to do with whether or not you can do the job rather than a letter of reference from a previous employer. A disagreement with one employer does not by any means make you unemployable. If you find you are getting job rejections and think it is because of your reference, then do ask to see a copy. You might find it is not the reference that is holding you back after all, but rather your lack of self-esteem, which might have been seriously dented through the negative experience of leaving your job. If this is the case, Part Two of this book explores ways in which this problem – one that is quite understandable – can be addressed and rectified. Then, with a decent reference and an even better attitude, there will be no stopping you!

PART TWO

What do I do now?

Although the world is full of suffering, it is also full of the overcoming of it.

Helen Keller (1880-1968)

4 TAKING ACTION

Imagine a group of people white-water rafting down the Zambezi River in Zambia when a dangerous eddy tips the raft and sends one member of the crew, a young woman, headlong into the foaming water. Despite wearing a life jacket she goes under for twenty seconds. When she emerges, gasping for breath, she discovers that her companions are nowhere in sight and that she is being swept swiftly downriver, glancing off rocks, logs and anything else that happens to be in her way.

Ahead of her in the river looms a large boulder. As the current dashes her into it, she manages to grasp the sharp, slippery surface. She is scared, exhausted and bruised – but, for the moment, safe. There is still no sign of her companions. But the riverbank is a tantalising ten feet to her right, separated from her by the surging current.

As she catches her breath, she considers her options. Should she stay clinging to the rock? She can probably last for another five or ten minutes at most before the cold water numbs and weakens her. Will the rescuers arrive before then? Or should she strike out for shore while she still has a little strength left in her arms and legs? If she leaves the safety of the boulder, will she be dragged under by the current and drowned? Time is of the essence. Her grip is slipping. What should she do?

One of the hardest things to do if you are suffering from work-related stress is deciding what action to take and when. As we have seen from Chapter Two, the longer you experience stress, the more likely you are to suffer physical, psychological and behavioural reactions, all of which can seriously affect your ability to take action and make changes. In time, you can actually find yourself too ill or tired to make any decisions at all, and you therefore remain trapped in a deplorable situation.

There is a grim paradox here. By the time you know that you must take action to relieve your stress, you are often incapable of doing so due to fatigue or illness. Ideally you need to be sufficiently self-aware and able to recognise when a situation is not right and starting to cause stress. Try to take action, in other words, before the uncongenial work situation drags you down with it – before you get swept away by the raging Zambezi River.

Choosing how to respond

How many times have you heard someone say, 'I have no choice'. One of the most demoralising aspects of being a victim is this sense of powerlessness – the feeling that we have no choice in our lives, that we are completely controlled and dominated by others. But this is a destructive – and ultimately wrong-headed – way of thinking. The point is that we do have a choice in how we respond to any situation that presents itself in life, though this choice is not always clear-cut nor the consequences risk-free.

It is difficult to imagine a power relationship more one-sided and grotesque than that found in the Nazi concentration camps during World War II. Yet even here, as Victor Frankl found, there was a certain freedom of choice among the inmates. Frankl survived over three years in four different concentration camps. After his release, he continued in his profession as a psychiatrist, building on his experiences from the camp to help other survivors. In his book, *Man's Search for Meaning*, first published in 1946, he writes of the camps: 'There were always choices to make. Every day, every hour, offered the opportunity to make a decision, a decision which determined whether you would or would not submit to those powers which threatened to rob you of your very self, your inner freedom; which determined whether or not you would become the plaything of circumstance, renouncing freedom and dignity to become moulded into the form of the typical inmate.'[1]

Therefore, if it is possible for concentration camp victims, under extreme physical and psychological stress, to make a decision – for example, to be compassionate to their fellow inmates – we too can make a decision as to how we respond to work-related stress. We must learn to take personal responsibility in alleviating the cause of our stress. In some situations, the solution might be to do nothing for the moment, whilst in other circumstances challenging a person or removing ourselves from the scene might be the appropriate course. The point is that, no matter how terrible our situation, we still have the power to make decisions – something that no one can take away.

First steps

Life shrinks or expands in proportion to one's courage.

Anais Nin (1903-1977)

There is no right or wrong way to proceed. Circumstances will vary, of course, depending on the nature and cause of the stress. However, there are many possible avenues to explore in order to find solutions to the causes of your work-related stress. There are many people – like line managers, counsellors, union officials – whose job it is to deal with the sort of problems you've been experiencing. It is important, therefore, to make the most of them. Remember – you are not alone!

Personnel and line managers

Excessive workloads, personal problems, threat of redundancy – all of these fall into the lap, in the first instance, of the line manager. In a healthy and supportive relationship, your line manager can often assist you in working out the best strategy for dealing with your problems. However, this is not always possible, because it may be your line manager who is causing your stress in the first place! In fact, two separate polls have suggested that some 50% of workers in Britain and Ireland believe they have a manager like David Brent, the 'boss from hell' in BBC's *The Office;* and a survey of 10,000 British men aged 18-44 found that bosses topped their lists of the biggest irritations in life – ahead of annoying partners, speed cameras and overpriced drinks.[2]

This rather bleak view of office relations is confirmed by another study. After interviewing 3,500 employees, Dr Patrick Gilbert, head of research at Mercer Human Resources, found that 24% of middle managers and 17% of senior managers reported in 2002 that they had been victims of bullying. Gilbert is alarmed about the high rate of bullying amongst managers because, as he points out, 'if managers are the victims of bullying, they are more likely to bully the people they manage'.[3]

In circumstances where talking to your line manager is inappropriate, it is advisable to make an appointment with either your personnel department or a senior manager. In organisations such as hospitals, county councils and universities, the personnel department can be quite large. Your section or department will probably be assigned a personnel officer who is responsible for you, and who should be your first port of call.

Personnel officers are usually university graduates with a background in human resources management, business management, social administration or psychology. These days most personnel officers will have the professional qualification – The Professional Development Scheme (PDS) administered by the Chartered Institute of Personnel and Development (CIPD) – and promotion is rare without such qualifications. Training for the qualification can take a year on a full-time course or three years part-time. 68% of CIPD members are female.

Duties as a personnel officer will vary according to the organisation but are likely to include:

- helping line managers to understand and implement the organisation's policies and procedures
- liaising with a wide range of organisations involved in areas such as race relations, disability, gender and health and safety
- recruiting staff: developing job descriptions, preparing advertisements, checking application forms, short listing candidates, interviewing and selecting

- developing policies on issues such as working conditions, performance management, equal opportunities, disciplinary procedures and absence management
- advising on pay and remuneration awards
- undertaking salary reviews
- administering payroll and maintaining records relating to staff
- interpreting and advising on employment legislation
- planning and sometimes delivering training
- implementing disciplinary procedures

Unfortunately, as Sally discovered, this person, despite full qualifications, is not always as helpful or objective as one would hope. Her manager, Moira, had written down a list of all Sally's alleged misdemeanours and called an unexpected meeting to read them out to her – what amounted, she recalls, to a litany of abuse. These included things as petty as the fact she was seen reading the newspaper at 4 pm. Sally was completely shocked by the triviality of it all, but she was also afraid of the malicious intentions behind Moira's behaviour. 'I kept breaking down in tears when I tried to explain to Personnel what was said and how it was broached,' Sally remembers. 'I was so upset I couldn't think straight, and it all came out like a silly child's account. I could see his eyes glaze over as he occasionally glanced at his watch. I left his office feeling even more abused.'

It should also be noted that small organisations might not have a personnel department. In these circumstances, it may be appropriate to talk to someone senior to your line manager. If at all possible, communication with someone in your organisation is the best course of action in the first instance. Nothing will change if no-one is aware of the problem. Crucially, you can insist that the first meeting is off the record and confidential.

Action points:

1. If appropriate, talk to your line manager. Go prepared with a written list of concerns.
2. If this is not appropriate, talk to your manager's own line-manager.
3. If you do not feel satisfied with the response, make an appointment to talk to someone in personnel.
4. You can request that meetings are, in the first instance, confidential and un-recorded. This shows that you are serious in finding a solution and not merely being confrontational with unrealistic demands.
5. Be very clear from the outset what you hope to achieve. If the purpose of your meeting is to complain about your bullying manager, be sure to give examples of his or her behaviour and what you expect should be done about it.

6. Often it is difficult to remain calm and unemotional when voicing concerns that have been bothering you for a while, but if at all possible try to remain so. If you do break down and cry, remember that tears are a common symptom of stress and should trigger a warning signal to the listener.

7. If you have advance warning of a scheduled meeting to discuss your concerns, practice beforehand in front of a mirror what you plan to say. It really does help!

8. Remember you can ask for a union rep to be present at any meeting you have with personnel or your line-manager.

Counsellors

Some organisations have access to counsellors, and it might be useful to talk to one in order to get your own ideas straight. A good counsellor will guide you into learning more about yourself and help to build up your self-esteem if it has been dented. He or she will also assist you with organising your thoughts and deciding what action, if any, needs to be taken. A registered counsellor who divulges any information about you without your consent will be struck off from their official body, the British Association for Counselling and Psychotherapy (BACP), so there should be no concern about secrets falling into the wrong hands.

It is important though to get the right counsellor for you and your circumstances, as there are many different schools of thought and approaches. There are some counsellors for example, who specialise in work-related stress and bullying, and your doctor, personnel department or occupational nurse can advise you on who is appropriate.

Any counsellor you choose should be fully accredited by the BACP, which means he or she will have completed a minimum of 250 hours of theory and 450 hours supervised practice plus some personal therapy. In fact, therapists are required to talk through their own issues with a qualified supervisor even when qualified.

Christine went to see one of the university counsellors of her own volition when she found that she simply couldn't cope with the overwhelming workload. She was new to the job as marketing officer and wanted to talk to someone in confidence about how she should deal with her situation. 'To be honest, I wish I had gone to speak to her earlier,' she now says, 'because I only had one session before I was forced to take sick leave.'

Christine had ignored the numbness in her arms and legs as it would come and go, but her body was in such a high state of stress alert that her nerve endings were actually becoming damaged. So impressed was she with the one session that she did have with the counsellor that she is convinced she might have been able to prevent her physical breakdown by having the confidence to confront her line manager before the situation got out of control.

However, not everyone is so impressed by counsellors. Margaret was discriminated against in her job as a information assistant because she had a back problem that was made worse by lifting and stacking books. 'It was my occupational nurse who recommended that I talk to someone. As my employer would be paying, I thought I'd give it a go.' Margaret was not impressed. 'I thought it was "money for old rope". To me the situation was clear-cut. My boss was insisting I stack and lift books. My doctor and occupational nurse stated this was damaging my health but the counsellor wanted to talk about my relationship with my mother and my attitude regarding authority. After two sessions I stopped going as I did not find this very helpful.'

For information about counsellors talk to your doctor, union, or occupational nurse, and refer to Helpful Contacts at the end of this book.

Action points:

1. Take time to find the right counsellor for you. Listen to recommendations from your doctor, union or occupational nurse. Do your own research by searching the web or Yellow Pages for local practitioners.
2. Make sure the counsellor is suitably qualified.
3. If after one or two sessions you are not comfortable with your counsellor, find another or simply stop attending. Counsellors are there to help you, but if they are not or are making you feel even worse, then they are not right for you.
4. Do not be afraid to discuss anything in your life that might not seem relevant to your current problem. A skilled counsellor will find links if there are any.
5. No-one at work other than your occupational nurse need know you are having counselling. When recording in advance any absences during work time, you need only say it is for a medical appointment.

The Union

Complain to one who can help you.

Yugoslav proverb

In 1999 the Employment Relations Act required that employers with at least twenty-one workers had to recognise their employees' right to have union representation if requested. However, according to the TUC (Trades Union Congress), 5.4 million employees are currently working in establishments with less than nineteen staff. That amounts to 21.8% of the UK workforce.[4] Therefore, turning to a union for help and support when experiencing work-related stress is not a realistic option for over twenty percent of the UK workforce.

Fortunately, large organisations like educational establishments or medical institutions might have one or two unions operating within the organisation. Staff at all levels can pay a monthly subscription to become a member, and this subscription is dependent on their salary. In return, a member can receive certain benefits ranging from reduced insurance policies and vacation offers to legal help and representation if required.

Union representatives are volunteers who are voted in by the members and can assist staff at work in disputes with employers. The Union pays the employer for the reps' time and also trains them, keeping them up to date with employment law and regulations. However, as the job is essentially voluntary, the service and support a member can expect will obviously vary. This is what John, a Careers Officer in his mid forties, discovered. 'I thought my union rep was completely useless,' John explained. 'He, like all of us, was worried about redundancy and didn't want to rock the boat. So he often watered down our complaints and concerns when talking to management.'

On the other hand, both Christine and Sally found their union representatives extremely helpful. 'I'm not sure how I would have coped without my rep,' Sally said. 'Both Personnel and Moira's line manager just didn't want to know, but my union rep could see by the evidence I produced that I was being systematically undermined and bullied. I don't know where I would have been without her.'

It was Sally's union representative who negotiated a satisfactory exit package. Christine's union representative set up and chaired meetings with personnel and her line manager, helping to work out strategies for reducing her workload. Both Christine and her line manager were relieved that this intervention was orchestrated by an independent person outside the department, which meant that personality differences were removed from the equation.

If work relations get to the point of irreconcilable differences, the union can help you to take a case to an industrial tribunal. This action is something that should not be undertaken lightly as the added stress it can cause, not to mention the financial losses that can be incurred, need serious consideration. For further information about unions, talk in the first instance to your personnel department and refer to Helpful Contacts at the end of this book.

Action points:

1. If you are not already a member of a union, check with colleagues or personnel whether any operate within your organisation.
2. After researching the most appropriate union for you – if there is more than one – contact your departmental union rep and join. Fees will be automatically deducted from your monthly pay cheque. If you feel your

departmental union rep is not as helpful as you would like, contact another outside the department.

3. Take to your first meeting examples and evidence of your work concerns.
4. Make notes of any meetings you have with your union rep for future reference if needed.

Keeping records

Those that cannot remember the past are condemned to repeat it.

George Santayana (1863-1952)

In the case of bullying, work overload, or the threat of redundancy, keeping records of meetings, conversations and incidents is always useful. When presenting a case, you need evidence. Without evidence it can be difficult for anyone to argue your point.

As we have seen in Chapter Two, memory loss and lack of concentration can be direct results of stress. Therefore it is all the more important to record incidents immediately after they happen, even if you are the sole witness. The time and energy that is spent on keeping a journal is enormous for both employer and employee, but on reflection, when re-read, these records show patterns and may be used as evidence in tribunals.

Sally had been advised by her union representative to keep a work diary, which she did daily. 'It took me a while to cotton on that I must record everything just as my manager was doing about me,' Sally said. 'It seemed so ridiculous. But thank goodness I did. I couldn't prove that I was not reading the newspaper at 4 pm, but I could prove that I was still in the office on the day she accused me of leaving early.'

Steve also found keeping a work diary useful, but for different reasons. 'It wasn't exactly a work diary, but I kept a journal at night and recorded conversations and events of the day. I never re-read anything until the careers adviser I saw suggested it. She suggested that I write down all the things that I didn't want from a job and I was able to see this clearly from my journal. It was really useful when deciding what to do next with my life.'

Action points:

1. Keep a notepad handy and write down any interactions that concern you. Make sure you date and time any entries.
2. Even if the situation looks as though it is sorting itself out, carry on recording events. In the case of bullying, it is not unusual for attacks to resume after a period of relative calm.
3. Keep copies of any written communication or emails you have with your co-workers or manager.

4. Keep your personal opinions about work safely away from the office and never write anything negative about the establishment or your co-workers in an email. Emails at work are not confidential.

5. Make sure that if you are absent from your desk or office you can account for your whereabouts. If there is no office diary in which to record such incidents, buy one yourself and record in advance every meeting, appointment or out-of-office event that you are likely to attend. Leave it in a public place on your desk.

6. Any request you make - for example to take leave or to attend a doctor's appointment – should be done by email and a copy made.

7. Any request made of you, especially a verbal one, should be responded to in writing. Keep a record. It sounds very petty, but in the case of bullying you can bet your bully is doing the same with you!

Occupational health

Advice is like snow; the softer it falls, the longer it dwells upon, and deeper it sinks into the mind.

Samuel Taylor Coleridge (1772-1834)

If you are suffering from work-related stress, your employer or doctor might recommend that you speak to an occupational nurse. Those on long-term sick leave might be required by their organisation to make an appointment with the occupational nurse on their return. This can be useful in order to talk through any concerns or worries. However, for some people, like Mark, a deputy retail store manager, this visit can initially be a worrying experience. 'Personnel suggested I speak to the occupational nurse,' he says, 'but my first reaction was, what good will that do? He is employed by the organisation that is condoning my bullying manager.'

Christine, too, felt anxious when on returning to work after several months off on sick leave, she was told it was standard practice at her university for a returnee to talk to the occupational nurse. 'I kept thinking she'd tell my boss that I was still on anti-depressants. I really didn't want anyone to know about that'.

The Nursing and Midwifery Council (NMC) is very aware of the fear that some people have about confidential information on themselves being leaked and ending up in the wrong hands. To reassure the public, the NMC state in their code of Professional Practice (2202) the following professional and ethical obligations for nurses:

To trust another person with private and personal information about yourself is a significant matter. If the person to whom that information is given is a nurse, midwife or health visitor, the patient or client has a right to believe that this information, given in confidence, will only be used for the purposes for which it was given and will not be released to others without their permission. The death of a patient or client does not give you the right to break confidentiality.[5]

So what exactly does an occupational nurse do? As a consequence of legislation, all businesses and organisations will either have their own health and safety adviser or they will pay a freelance expert for their services. It is these professionals who are responsible for creating, maintaining and improving health and safety within the work place. They ensure that all safety legislation is adhered to and that the workplace is therefore a safe environment. Health and Safety advisers should be corporate members of The Institution of Occupational Safety and Health (IOSH) and have an MSc/ postgraduate diploma in Occupational Safety and Health, an accredited degree in occupational health and safety, or the National Examination Board for Occupational Safety and Health (NEBOSH) diploma. Occupational nurses are often part of the health and safety team of an organisation, but their qualifications and expertise come from a different perspective.

Occupational nurses are well qualified and on top of their basic nursing training they will have taken extra courses to qualify professionally in this area of specialisation. Many have also had experience of working in an accident and emergency setting as this is deemed particularly useful experience. Occupational nurses have an important role in the work place and are responsible for:

- The prevention of health problems, promotion of healthy living and working conditions.
- Understanding the effects of work on health and health at work.
- Basic first aid and health screening
- Workforce and workplace monitoring and health need assessment.
- Health promotion.
- Education and training.
- Counselling and support.
- Risk assessment and risk management.

Although occupational nurses are employed by the organisation that is causing your work-related stress, they should act independently of their employer and advise and support you in your response to the situation. They can only disclose information about you without your consent if they think you are a danger to yourself or work colleagues. This, in practice, is very rare, and the occupational nurse would have to ensure his or her reasons were well supported by documentary evidence.

The occupational nurse can refer you to a counsellor if he/she thinks it could be helpful. Sometimes counselling is paid for by your employer and unless you tell anyone you are seeing a counsellor, it will remain confidential and your boss will not know. If the occupational nurse thinks it could support your case, he/she might suggest you sign a form giving him/her permission to write to your doctor, who can confirm you are suffering from stress. However, the occupational nurse cannot do this without your consent. The downside of this option is that the information will be stored by your employer – although they cannot have access to it without your consent – for eight to ten years.[6] Records made under the 1988 Control of Substances Hazardous to Health Regulations means information in certain circumstances, is stored for forty years.

The upside of agreeing to obtain a doctor's report is that the occupational nurse can use this information to help you negotiate a financial settlement or compensation if the case is taken to a tribunal. However you need to ask yourself whether it will help you to achieve the outcome you want. If it is unlikely to assist, then do not sign the consent form.[7] Moreover your doctor will charge for this service, and in some situations it is you, and not your employer, who will be presented with the bill. The cost can vary, but on average it is in the region of £70. It is therefore in your interest to check at the outset who will pay. If you decide to go ahead with this option, you can also tick the box on the consent form confirming that you would like to read the doctor's letter before it is sent to the occupational nurse. This option will delay the process for several weeks but might give you peace of mind. However, even if you do not see the report before it leaves the doctor's office, you still have the right of access to it for six months after its release.[8]

As the law is clear regarding how information about you can be used and distributed, you have nothing to fear when talking to an occupational nurse. Should they divulge any information that you have not agreed in advance, it could mean litigation and the loss of their career. Talking to this professional can be helpful, as he or she will no doubt be able to offer constructive advice on how to alleviate your stress. In the wider picture, informing them of problems in the work place assists them in making it a safer environment for all employees. A good occupational nurse is an extremely valuable resource to both the employer and employee.

Action points:

1. If it has not already been mentioned, enquire whether it is possible to talk to an occupational nurse.
2. Only agree for the occupational nurse to request a health report from your doctor if you think it will help your case.
3. If you agree to a doctor's health report, confirm who will pay the fee. If you are expected to cover the costs, decide whether it will be worth it in the long run.
4. Tick the box requesting to see the doctor's health report before it leaves

the surgery. You can request to have it changed or facts omitted if you prefer.

5. Think in advance how you want the occupational nurse to help you. If there are sufficient grounds, he or she can build a case against your employer or negotiate with your manager on your behalf, and can even conduct a risk assessment on your particular job. So be clear in you own mind as to what outcome you hope to achieve.

Taking time out

The man who is swimming against the stream knows the strength of it.

Woodrow Wilson (1856-1924)

Prolonged stress, as we have seen, can cause a range of physical, psychological and behavioural symptoms. Therefore, for some people, removing themselves physically from the cause of their stress – that is, their work place – perhaps by taking sick leave, is the only way to move forward.

Sick leave may be obtained only under specific conditions, and you will need a doctor's certificate for any time off longer than seven days. This means a trip to your GP, that invaluable resource for stressed-out workers. This visit can often be a crucial one. Sally became so fraught after months of being bullied and undermined in her job as a physiotherapist that in desperation she made an appointment to see her GP. Her doctor was extremely sympathetic and immediately recognised that Sally needed time away from the work place. At first Sally was appalled at the suggestion and initially rejected her idea. 'Looking back, I can't believe I actually sat there arguing with my GP when she suggested signing me off for two weeks. I kept saying that I was too busy to take time out. It was totally irrational – I was not sleeping, I was having panic attacks and I was completely exhausted. And yet I still wanted to go back to work! '

Sally eventually took four months off on full pay. For six of those weeks she slept excessively and felt generally unwell. 'It wasn't until about two months into my sick leave that I started to comprehend what I'd been through. With help from a counsellor I was then ready to start reassessing my working life. Having time out gave me the space, free from office pressures, to do this.'

Fay, who is in her early forties, was also thankful for the intervention of her GP. She had experienced the death of six of her close friends and family in just five years, and was struggling to cope with a mortgage on her own after a divorce. She returned to education after her marriage ended and eventually managed to secure an interesting job in the archives department of a local council in Somerset. The only catch, of course, was that she was on a temporary contract. On the last day of her final temporary contract – and after months of debilitating physical symptoms – Fay walked into her doctor's surgery, demanding to see her GP. She felt almost suicidal with despair.

Without an appointment, she was seen by her doctor, who immediately put her on anti-depressants and signed her off on sick leave. He did this despite her contract coming to an end so she would not be pressurised by Social Security to look for work. Her doctor recognised that she needed time out to rest and heal. It took Fay six months to get well enough to work again and, like Sally, she spent the first month simply sleeping.

Dr Simon Fradd, chairman of the Doctor Patient Partnership (DPP), says that stress is the second biggest cause of sick leave for employees in the UK. To counteract the problem, the DPP launched a campaign in 2003 to raise awareness of stress related problems with employers, producing a leaflet entitled *A Note to Employers* which employees can obtain from their GPs. Part of the reasoning behind this campaign, says Dr Fradd, is the enormous pressure that is put upon GPs for stress-related care and treatment. 'It is up to us all as individuals, employers and society to place the highest possible premium on looking after our minds. The figures associated with not doing so speak for themselves.'[9] One of these figures is particularly alarming: a survey by Pulse and BBC One's *Now You're Talking!* found that GPs themselves are casualties of stress, with four in five of them reporting symptoms.[10]

Nevertheless, if, like Sally or Fay, you need time out to heal, then talking to your GP is absolutely essential. As Sally's doctor tried to explain to her, taking time out away from the office would in the long term be more beneficial to her overall well-being – and that of her employer as well – than struggling on with no respite. 'I could only make those important decisions about my future,' says Sally, 'after having time to recharge my batteries in a safe environment away from work. My doctor was one hundred percent on the right track in her diagnosis.'

Do not be afraid, therefore, to talk to your doctor about taking time out to heal and take stock. It is not a holiday, but time well spent in getting your body back in balance and working properly. In time, you will be ready to start researching your next move and rejoining the workforce. As the Roman poet Ovid once wrote, 'A field that has rested gives a bountiful crop.'

Action points:

1. Make an appointment to talk to your doctor. Your doctor will only sign you off on sick leave if he/she thinks it is necessary for your well-being.
2. Your doctor might suggest anti-depressants or sleeping pills. Ask what the side effects are and how long you can expect to be on medication.
3. Do your own research into the medication your doctor recommends by searching for information on the web.

4. If you feel your doctor is not sympathetic or is not really listening to your concerns, ask to see another one.

Family and close friends

Advice from your friends is like the weather, some of it good, some of it bad.

Anonymous

You can choose your friends, the saying goes, but you can't choose your family. Still, we have many reasons to be thankful for our families, because research has shown that they can help to keep us healthy. Numerous studies indicate good relationships and strong family support networks influence health for the better. A classic study concerns the town of Roseto, an Italian-American community in Pennsylvania, the inhabitants of which were studied for over fifty years. Initially the researchers found the population of Roseto experienced extremely low mortality rates from heart attacks in comparison to neighbouring towns. By the late 1960s and early 1970s, however, the death rate due to heart attacks rose, and the researchers concluded that Roseto had shifted from the three-generation household with strong commitments to religion and relationships to a less cohesive, fragmented and isolated community similar to their neighbouring towns.[11] This trend is not limited to Roseto. A study of 7,000 men and women in Alameda County, near San Francisco, concluded that those who lacked social ties – friends, family, marriage, church or group membership – were 1.9 to 3.1 times more likely to die during a ten-year period than those enjoying more traditional and mutually supporting families and groups.[12]

There is no question that having a support network of family and close friends, can be beneficial when you are working through a crisis. Not only will your general sense of wellbeing be nurtured, but your physical health, according to these studies, will be protected from 'dis-eases'.[13]

Still, there are limits to what your family can do for you – and some caveats as well. Talking ideas and options over with family and close friends can be useful, but remember that when discussing anything that involves yourself, you must be the one to make the final decision. It is surprising how many of us give away our decision-making powers. Sometimes it seems easier to have someone else make the choice for us – not least because we can then blame them if things go wrong! However, you need to learn not to be afraid to take responsibility for any decisions that you make. After all, we learn from our mistakes. How else would a small child who touches the hot stove learn not to barbecue his fingers in future?

Don't forget how important a social support system can be, but be aware that some family and close friends, no matter how well-meaning, may have no conception of what you are experiencing – and consequently they can give the wrong advice. Christine's father was appalled when she told him she was to take several months off recuperating on sick leave. He tried hard to dissuade her from doing so, as he was worried that this would affect her long-term career prospects. Fortunately, Christine did not take his advice and was able to recover from stress and exhaustion before returning refreshed to the workforce.

Likewise, Steve's parent's ignored his frustration and blatant lethargy, repeatedly reminding him how lucky he was to have a job. His parents were also well-meaning in their comments, but they were from a different generation with an attitude coloured by their experience of unemployment and poverty. To them any job was better than no job at all. Both Christine and Steve, however, were the first to admit how comforting it was to have family members around or at the end of a phone, as it helped them feel that they were not totally alone and isolated during a stressful episode in their lives.

Margaret, similarly, took her friend's advice and went to see a solicitor about her appalling situation at work. 'My friend encouraged me to do so because I was being asked to do a job that was not in my job description and it was damaging my health. My friend even came with me to the first session. I'm not sure,' Margaret said, 'if I would have had the courage to go on my own.'

The next chapter will explore what options are available to you as a victim of stress: leaving your job, moving sideways, re-training and gaining further skills, or downshifting. It will also offer you practical advice on how to do this. In the meantime, you might find it useful to answer the following questions.

Action points:

1. What are the circumstances of the person who is giving advice? Are they happily married, unhappily divorced, employed, retired, content with their life etc?
2. Do you aspire to their lifestyle? If not, they may not be the right person to advise you, as their opinions are likely to be coloured by their own experiences and perspectives.
3. Never ask someone, 'what would you do?' and then blindly follow their advice without considering all the options.
4. Write down on separate pieces of paper the advice and opinions of all those who offer advice. Then write down what solution you ideally would like to see. How similar are the views?
5. Are you someone who always wants to please others or has difficulty in saying no. If yes to either question counselling or self-esteem support groups or courses might be particularly useful to you.

5 SHOULD I STAY OR SHOULD I GO?

How many people – not just those suffering from work-related stress – have dreamt of saying to their boss something like what the American country and western artist Johnny Paycheck sang in 1978?

Take this job and shove it,
I ain't workin' here no more.

But before you follow the example of Paycheck's harassed worker and do anything rash, it is sensible to take a deep breath, step back and reassess your options. You have already taken the first steps by choosing to face up to your stress. Now it's time to plan what to do about it. Can you stay in the job and make it work for you? Or is leaving and finding other employment a better option? It's the old dilemma faced by anyone who finds himself caught between an uncomfortable situation, on the one hand, and a completely unknown one on the other. Should I stay or should I go?

Reassessing

Ralph Waldo Emerson once wrote, 'Finish each day and be done with it. You have done what you could; some blunders and absurdities have crept in; forget them as soon as you can. Tomorrow is a new day; you shall bring it serenely and with too high a spirit to be encumbered with your old nonsense.' Although on the one hand these are wise words – why carry your old nonsense with you? – it is sometimes extremely useful to look back over yesterday's challenges in order to prevent similar mistakes occurring tomorrow. One way of doing this is to reassess your situation, either alone with pen and paper or, if preferred, with the help of a professionally qualified careers adviser.

Careers advice

A careers adviser is someone who, along with your GP and counsellor, may be able to throw you a life-line if your stress is so severe that the only option for you is to consider abandoning ship. For many people, talking to a careers adviser or consultant can be extremely useful when they are making major changes in their working life. Careers advisers are not counsellors, though some also might have counselling qualifications. Most will have a degree plus further relevant qualifications to certificate, diploma or MA standards. In addition, many careers advisers have experience in recruitment and training in the professions, commerce and industry, lending breadth to their knowledge.

What can you expect if you make an appointment to see a careers adviser? You will be offered impartial advice on a one-to-one basis and helped to explore ideas about your goals in life, no matter how whimsical or unrealistic they may seem. As with doctors, counsellors and occupational therapists, your meeting with a careers adviser remains confidential. A careers adviser might also suggest that you take a psychometric test (on which more later) to assist you in learning more about your personal qualities and aptitudes, and therefore about what career might suit you. Some of these tests are computer-based but others are taken in exam conditions. For the latter, the careers adviser must be qualified at least to Level A of the British Psychological Association's standards, and often to the higher Level B. On top of that, there is a further week-long training course in the administration of psychometric tests.

Let us follow the case of Steve, the economics graduate who found after two years that work as a researcher at a London borough council was so tedious and soul-destroying that it actually made him ill. If, like Steve, you are a recent graduate, you can return to your university within three years of graduation and receive free careers advice. Any UK graduate within this three-year time frame can also visit any other university careers centre and request careers advice. However, graduates from a university other than their own are usually charged a small one-off fee of between five and twenty pounds for this service.

For graduates outside the time-frame, as well as for non-graduates, there are several other options for receiving careers advice. In the first instance it is worth contacting IAG (Information, Advice and Guidance), a network of adult guidance organisations.[1] The IAG will provide information on the whereabouts of local advice centres, and some will offer their services for free, only charging a fee for psychometric testing. If you prefer, there is also a range of private careers consultants you can contact. They will charge for their services and can sometimes be quite expensive, but in addition to guidance and psychometric testing they also offer support with the job application process, and some have direct contacts with employers. Contact numbers and addresses can be found in your local yellow pages or on the internet. If you do not want face-to-face contact with a careers adviser, there are countless careers web sites that offer free psychometric tests, careers information and CV packages. To find these, use one of the numerous search engines on the web.

With the guidance of a careers adviser from his former university, Steve not only learnt more about himself and what he liked and disliked about his job, but he also found a new career path that suited him much better. The careers adviser wanted

Steve to examine his present situation before looking at alternatives. She therefore asked him to write down his answers to the following questions – ones of relevance to any employees re-examining their careers or, more generally, their goals in life.

Question one: What is your job title?
Researcher in the economic planning department of a London Borough Council.

Question two: Why did you apply for this post?
Because it was convenient. It was located near my parent's house, enabling me to move in with them and not pay rent. This meant I could repay my student debts.

Question three: What aspects do you like about this job?
- working on a project from beginning to end
- contributing information to developing policy
- researching, preparing and writing reports
- working with members of the public, specialists, councillors and external agencies

Question four: What aspects do you dislike about this job?
- my co-workers
- time drags
- not being allowed to use my initiative
- criticism from my boss
- repetitive tasks

Question five: What would others say you naturally do well?
- I bring enthusiasm to a project
- I'm good with numbers
- I'm tenacious

Question six: What do you do in your spare time?
- play tennis
- read widely (novels, newspapers, biographies)
- watch telly (especially historical and current affairs documentaries)
- used to be a volunteer fund-raiser for a charity providing UK holidays for underprivileged children.

Question seven: What cause(s) do you feel strongly about?
- Freedom of speech
- Human rights for everyone

Question eight: How would you like to be remembered?
- As someone who combined doing something good for others with being able to earn a living.
- As someone who made the most of his days and didn't waste his life.

Question nine: What accomplishments in your life have meant the most to you?
- Getting my swimming badge in Scouts when I hated the water.
- Managing to fund-raise over £7,000 for Children in Need whilst studying for my university finals.
- Spending four weeks as a volunteer one summer at a holiday camp for underprivileged children. Not only was it brilliant fun, but it was so rewarding to see how happy the kids were doing things like abseiling, pot-holing and camping out – things they would never otherwise have had the opportunity to experience.

Question ten: What would you choose to do if you were not concerned about time or money?
- Work for a charity as a volunteer in a Third World country.
- Work with like-minded people.
- Travel

Steve knew he was in the wrong job, but it now became clearer to him why it was stressing him so much. Putting aside the obvious – that he took the job because of convenience and the ability to pay off his student debts – he began to understand more about himself and what he wanted from life.

By taking the time to reassess, Steve discovered that he likes to work with people but prefers to feel part of a like-minded team. He likes to get his teeth into a project and doesn't enjoy being bored or doing repetitive tasks. He can be enthusiastic and tenacious in the right situation, has a strong sense of the unfairness of the world, and wants to contribute to making it a better place, for example, by helping people. He is obviously someone who has shown much initiative in the past and is undaunted by taking on challenges. Analysing all of this information with his careers adviser, Steve was able to see how he needed to make some drastic career changes to achieve his full potential in the world of work.

Answering questions similar to those above is one way of reassessing your present situation. Another way is by taking a psychometric test. The term 'psychometric' sounds a little off-putting. However, the 'psycho' in psychometric has nothing to do with shower scenes in Alfred Hitchcock films: it means 'of the mind', while 'metric' simply means 'measurement'. So the psychometric test is merely a measurement of your mind – a means of discovering your likes, dislikes and abilities. Psychometric tests or exercises are used to determine whether or not you have the specific abilities or personal qualities required for a particular job. There are two main types of tests: Aptitude (which measures your reasoning capabilities - verbal, numerical and spatial) and Personality (how and why you act and behave, your attitudes and preferences).

Unlike an aptitude test, you cannot fail a personality test. There is no 'right' or 'wrong' personality type! There are, however, preferred personality types for particular jobs, and this is why employers often use such tests. For example, in any given team there may be several personality types who are similar – people who are perfectionists and like to finish tasks before starting new ones. A manager might want the next team member to be someone who is capable of seeing the overall picture and can complete several tasks at the same time. In this way, a team can have a balance of skills. If you are thinking of a career change, it is definitely worth experimenting with a careers psychometric test because included in the results is a list of careers that might suit you, some of which you may not have even have considered before.

Similar to a counsellor, then, a careers adviser will help you to identify your strengths and weaknesses, and in addition will be able to suggest a job that might suit your particular talents. Whatever your needs, remember that you are not alone. There is always a solution to your work-place dilemma – you might just need a bit of help from an impartial careers professional in finding it.

A man with a plan

Writing Action Plans became fashionable in the early 1990s when nearly every Year 11 pupil in the UK was presented with an Action Plan that summarized their career aspirations. Compulsory action planning was soon dropped; it was simply too early for many 16-year olds realistically to know what they wanted and many of them saw the process as a waste of time.

However, an Action Plan is just a fancy name for making a list of your goals and how you can reach them. It is a fluid document that can change as you research your ideas and get nearer to reaching your goal. It is a way of clarifying your ideas at a particular time in your life, and it is always interesting to look back over your past Action Plans and see how these have developed as you gain in experience and knowledge.

There are no hard and fast rules about how to write an Action Plan, but for it to be effective it needs to reflect your overall aim. That aim can be vague - such as finding a career that 'helps people' or a job that includes working with numbers. It can be fine-tuned at a later stage when you have more information available. Action Plans are most effective if they are split into two sections: Planning and Action. So let us take Steve's Action Plan as an example, bearing in mind that he had discussed many ideas first with a Careers Adviser and knew at this point that he was interested in a career working with charities.

ACTION PLAN

Name: Steve

Career aims:

1. To work abroad for a few months in a charity as a volunteer.
2. To find paid employment in a charity or non-governmental organisation in a professional capacity.

Planning (gathering the facts)

1. Research volunteer work abroad.
2. Research details, training and entry qualifications of careers in charities such as charity fundraiser, charity officer, public relations officer, training and development officer, accountant.
3. Refer to **www.prospects.ac.uk** (a graduate careers advisory web site) or visit the local library, local careers office or other careers sites on the web.

Action (implementing the plan)

1. Curriculum Vitae (CV): update.
2. Volunteer work abroad: Decide length of time and preferred location, availability of living expenses and/or personal cash required. If the latter, how will this be raised?
3. Charities: Send updated CV and covering letter to charities asking for volunteer work.
4. Timescale: Decide preferred starting time.
5. Training: Investigate options for further training, including timing and length of courses, and whether full, part-time or on-the-job study is available.
6. Finances: Discover training costs, availability of grants or bursaries, and possibility of obtaining a loan.
7. Further education: Make applications for training courses.
8. Review: check progress in 2 months.

Action planning is a useful tool to help you move forward, even if you stay in your present job. Relieving work-related stress does not always mean leaving your job, of course. It could involve working out a plan to reduce your workload or taking training courses that will give you the skills to cope better with your job. Writing an Action Plan will help you to clarify the options available and the steps required to follow these up. It can be a positive experience that will lead you in the right direction – perhaps even one that you hadn't previously considered.

Updating your CV

In 1482 a young jobbing artist from Florence named Leonardo da Vinci wrote a letter to the Duke of Milan. In this letter he outlined his many abilities: he was able, he claimed, to build bridges, dig underground tunnels, devise catapults and 'flame-throwing engines', sink enemy ships, and 'make covered vehicles, safe and unassailable, which will penetrate enemy ranks with their artillery and destroy the most powerful troops.'[2] He was available, he concluded, for a job interview: if the Duke so wished, he would demonstrate all and any of these deadly skills and inventions in His Lordship's park.

So Leonardo, who is often given credit for inventing the helicopter, the bicycle, the armoured tank and the submarine, also appears to have invented something equally useful: the Curriculum Vitae (CV). Leonardo aside, Mrs Sarah Massey is reputed to have created the first CVs for her business, 'Mrs Massey's Agency', which supplied domestic servants to the English aristocracy during the 1800s. In those days CVs were no more than character references and a list of previous employers and skills that had been acquired. Potential employers could then choose between the various CVs for interviewing. CVs as we now know them took off during the Second World War when large numbers of people were required to contribute to the war effort and a document outlining potential employee's skills was needed in order to place them in a suitable job.

If the solution to your work-related stress is finding another job, then high on your to-do list will be up-dating your own CV. There are three ways of finding a new job: answering an advertisement, writing to an employer on spec, and networking – which means using any contacts you might have in your search for employment. In all cases, a professional-looking CV is absolutely vital.

It is worth noting that an employer who uses an in-house application form when recruiting usually wants the candidate to have certain skills. The application form directs the candidate to give the employer specific information. However, employers who use CVs as opposed to application forms want different information. The candidate is given a free rein to express what he/she thinks is important for the job advertised. This is why a CV is so important; try to second-guess what the employer is looking for and never merely send out a standard CV. Always research the company and the job advertised before putting pen to paper (or fingers to the keyboard).

As with Action Plans, there are no carved-in-stone rules about writing a CV, though certain guidelines need to be followed. If you plan to write your own CV it is always useful to look at samples to get an idea of different layouts. Stylistically, CVs will vary depending on the market they are aimed at. For example, a CV for a law firm should be presented in a rather conservative style, whereas one for an advertising agency might be presented on brightly coloured paper or in unusual fonts to show the employer how creative you are. If unsure, however, it is always best to act on the conservative side when devising the lay-out of a CV as you do not know the tastes of the person reading it. Here are some general principles for writing a CV:

- Make a few drafts - and don't expect perfection on the first attempt.
- Always check and double check spelling and grammar.
- Get someone you trust to check your CV. Sometimes it is hard to see glaring mistakes yourself.
- Do not include anything unnecessary, and never repeat yourself.
- Your CV must be directed at the job you are applying for or the company you are writing to on spec. Make it relevant and specific. To do this, research the job or company beforehand.
- Do not send out a standard CV for every job you apply for and never send a CV to an employer without stating what you want. An employer will not have time to search for a job that might just suit you.
- Make sure the CV is no longer than two pages.
- It is not necessary to include your marital status, your date of birth or your gender, although if you have a name which might not make your gender obvious you might want to clarify this. If you are a UK or EU citizen you do not need to include your nationality, but many people still do in order that there is no confusion about their right to work in the UK.
- Most CVs are written chronologically starting with the most recent qualification or job and going backwards. Do not worry about including months, especially if you have had more than one job in any year.
- Though not essential, many CVs will include a Profile at their beginning. This is where you can write a couple of sentences outlining what you can offer and what you are looking for.
- Include details of your skills that you think relevant to the job or company to whom you are applying.
- Include a section on your achievements. Some employers regard this as extremely important even if you think it is not. For example, putting down that one of your achievements was completing a sponsored run and raising £350 for Cancer Research shows an employer that you have commitment, tenacity and integrity.
- If you are worried about your references you can put 'References supplied on request' or 'please contact me first before approaching my references'.
- More and more employers are accepting CVs via email, but if you do send one by post make sure it is laser-printed on good quality white or cream paper.
- Unless you are applying for an extremely creative position, use colour sparingly on a CV. For example, it might look classy with a navy border or

your name highlighted in the same colour, but anything too bright or too colourful will look, to most employers, tacky and unprofessional.

- Always enclose a covering letter, whether by post or email, telling the employer exactly why you are sending your CV and highlighting three or four reasons why you think you are a suitable person to employ.

As already explained there is no right or wrong way to write a CV, so let us take a look at an example, that of Steve.

Stephen Surname

1 The Street	☎ 0208 000 1111
The Town	☎ 0777 7777 77
London SW1 2BB	e-mailto:steve@hotmail.com

PROFILE

Confident researcher and report writer who likes to work in a team. Interested in pursuing a career in fund-raising for a non-governmental or charitable organisation. Extremely numerate with experience in this field.

STUDIES

1998 – 2001	University of Nottingham: Bsc Economics 2:1
1996 – 1998	St Thomas Comprehensive School, London, A'levels: Economics (A), Maths (B),History (B)
1991 – 1996	St Thomas Comprehensive School, London, GCSEs: 9 grades A and B including maths and English

RELEVANT WORK EXPERIENCE

2000 – 2001	Volunteer fund-raiser for **Children in Need**. Organised student events and supervised the collection of monies

WORK EXPERIENCE

2001 -	**London Borough Council,** Research Assistant in economic planning department. Duties include researching and writing draft reports and liaising with interested parties.
2001	**Welsh Holiday Camp,** Tennis coach (Volunteer) for underprivileged children sponsored by a charity.

1996 – 2001   Variety of part-time employments whilst studying in London and
               Nottingham:
               Sainsbury's check-out assistant, **All Bar One** bartender, **Esso** petrol
               station checkout assistant

SKILLS

IT Skills: Excel, Microsoft, Powerpoint, Typing 60 wpm
Languages: French (conversational)
Numerical: A'level Maths and degree level in economics
Communication skills: Gained working as checkout assistants, in a charity for chil-
               dren, and through fund-raising.
               Driving Licence: Clean

ACHIEVEMENTS

2001   Raised £7,000 for Children in Need
2000   Worked with underprivileged children from Liverpool in a holiday
               camp in Wales
1994   Achieved swimming badge for Scouts despite my fear of water

INTERESTS

Tennis (school and university teams and member of South London Lawn Tennis
Club), amateur rowing (university team), reading and films

REFERENCES

Mr Joe Bloggs   Mrs Jane Bloggs
London Borough Council   Welsh Holiday Camp
London   Wales
☎ 0207 000 0000   ☎ 01459 000 0000
Email: **Email:**
bloggs@londoncouncil.org.uk   **bloggs@charity.ac.uk**

As CVs can make or break your application, it is important that you spend time on
lay-out, format and, of course, content. The font should not be smaller than 12 point.
There are countless books to buy on the subject, and a number of web sites offer free
templates to copy. If you are in the slightest bit unsure of how best to present yourself, however, visit a professional careers adviser or CV specialist. You might not have

all of the astounding talents and skills of Leonardo da Vinci – who did, after all, get the post with the Duke of Milan – but aim to make your CV land on the desk of your prospective employer with the same can't-say-no self-confidence of his letter!

Money Matters

For some people the answer to alleviating work-related stress is to leave their job and try something completely different, such as down-shifting, retraining, setting up their own business, or even just reducing their working hours. But before getting carried away with enthusiasm you need to try injecting the hypodermic of realism into the balloon of your dreams. For instance, can you afford to finance your new initiative or will you need to take out a loan? Incurring debt can, if not properly managed, lead you into trouble and actually add to your stress levels, as the British Association for Counselling and Psychotherapy found in their annual survey of 2001/02. They discovered that large numbers of students visiting a counsellor in that period complained of the 'twin miseries of debt and poverty'[3]. Moreover, researchers at Ohio State University interviewed 1,036 people and found there was a link between owing money and increased stress, resulting in worsening health.[4] Finding yourself in debt, then, can send you hopping out of the proverbial fry pan and into the fire.

That much said, with some careful preparation and planning beforehand, the debt incurred for a change in your working life can be contained and managed. Step number 1 is to clarify your current monthly expenses. Step number 2 is to look at ways you can reduce your monthly outgoings. Step number 3 is to make a budget – and step number 4 is to stick to it!

Step 1: Monthly Expenditure.

One way of discovering exactly what your monthly expenditures are is to keep a note of everything you spend in a month. You will be amazed at how much you are splashing out on non-essentials – CDs, drinks, eating out, clothes, holidays and so forth. Discover what *your* weakness is!

Another constructive way to work out your monthly expenditure is to fill out a Personal Monthly Budget Planner. Sounding more complicated than it is, this is a very useful exercise for anyone intent on taking control of their personal finances. Below is a standard form that will help you to do this.

PERSONAL MONTHLY BUDGET PLANNER

LIST OF ITEMS	MONTHLY EXPENDITURE
Mortgage/rent	
Property maintenance	
Council tax	
House contents/ building insurance	
Water charges	
Coal/gas/heating	
Electricity	
Telephone	
Mobile telephone	
Life assurance	
Credit card payments	
Hire purchase payments	
Personal loan repayments	
Car licence	
Car insurance	
Petrol/oil/other car expenses	
TV licence	
TV rental	
Train/bus fares/season ticket	
Food/drink/housekeeping	
Clothing/shoes	
School uniforms	
School meals	
Club/society subscriptions	
Newspaper/magazine subscriptions	
Savings/commitments/investments	
Holiday expenses	
Presents/Christmas expenditure	
Other expenses	
TOTAL MONTHLY EXPENDITURE	

Step 2: Reducing Your Monthly Expenditure

Now look at these monthly outgoings and think what, realistically, you can cut back. Here are some ideas of how you can make savings.

1. *Compare Prices:* Short of moving out to cheaper lodgings, there is not much you can do about reducing your rent - but there is if you have a mortgage. Shop around and find a better mortgage deal. Some canny homeowners change their mortgage lenders every couple of years. Invest in *Which Magazine* for up-to-date information on the best mortgage deals. Shop

around also for the best deals on house contents and building insurances, credit cards and loans. Web sites worth taking a look at are **www.uswitch. com** for utility and phone comparisons; **www.unrarelit.com** for credit cards and loans comparisons; **www.buy.co.uk** for water utilities comparisons; and **www.moneysupermarket.com** for comparisons of banks.

2. *Direct Debit:* Around 16,000 organisations currently use direct debits, which are automatic monthly payments of bills. Most companies offer considerable discounts if you pay in this way - often as much as up to 13% off the original price. Knowing exactly how much is debited each month will make budgeting easier to plan. A useful resource to consult is the web site **www. directdebit.co.uk.**

3. *Buy online:* You often get very good deals if you buy goods and services online. It is worth checking the internet to see if it has cheaper deals than the High Street. Another advantage of on-line shopping is that you eliminate bus fares, petrol and parking.

4. *Double up:* Many utility or insurance suppliers offer a discount if you use more than one of their products, for example, combining gas and electric services. A little bit of research could save you pounds.

5. *Use less:* Check out **www.ukpower.co.uk** for tips on how to use less energy in the house. For example, you can get some deals where energy is cheaper to run through the night so it will cost less to run your washing machine between certain times. Also, learn to switch off lights and heating when you are not in the house and shut doors to keep out the draughts. There are so many little things you can do to conserve energy – habits that help the environment as well as your wallet.

6. *Telephone:* Sign up for a low cost international telephone provider, and make national phone-calls during off-peak hours, usually between 6pm and 8am, and at weekends. Don't use your mobile phone unless you have to for emergencies and switch to a pay-as-you-go deal rather than a monthly subscription.

7. *Food shopping:* We could all spend a little less on food without necessarily eating less, if we just took the time to plan meals and where we shop. Here are some tips for making savings to your food bills.

Tips:

- Never go food shopping when you are hungry.
- Avoid ready meals and takeaway foods. They are expensive and full of unhealthy additives.

- Cook simple dishes such as baked potatoes with fillings or pasta and stews.
- Make your own sandwiches or salads instead of buying readymade ones.
- Don't buy all your food at the large supermarkets; look for budget supermarkets and local shops.
- Buy vegetable produce at local markets or farms and get what is in season.
- Bulk-buy staples such as tinned tomatoes, baked beans, pasta and rice.
- Write a list of what you are going to buy when you go food shopping and stick to the list (unless you see an incredible bargain!).

If you find you have more time on your hands, why not consider growing your own vegetables in a patch in your garden? If you do not have a large enough garden, put your name down for an allotment. The average cost of renting an allotment is £10 a year. That certainly won't break the bank and getting involved with an allotment can be a way of meeting people, not to mention enjoying fresh vegetables and produce. And gardening is, of course, a wonderful way to relax.

Take in a lodger: This will not be possible for everybody, but if you have the room why not think of taking a lodger for a short time to help with the mortgage? If you don't like the idea of having someone in your home all the time, it sometimes is possible to offer lodgings Monday to Thursdays to someone who is working away from their home during the week. Alternatively, if you live near a theatre or playhouse you might be able to offer Bed and Breakfast for thespians during their run.

Step 3: Plan Your Monthly Budget

Now that you know your monthly outgoings and have found ways of cutting back on your expenditure, it is possible to plan a monthly budget. Add on 10% for any hidden extras like an unexpected birthday present, car expenses or a broken washing machine. This budget is the minimum that you can live on per month. The next question is – can you afford to, and if you can't, should you take a loan to finance your change in lifestyle?

Bank Loans: Be extremely cautious about taking a loan to cover expenses when starting up your own business or re-training, and always do your homework first. Read the small print and be clear how much you will have to repay and when. Never be tempted to borrow money from a 'loan shark': unregulated interest repayment charges will only add to your existing stress levels and in some cases you may even lose your property if you cannot deliver the repayments on time.

Re-training

As the ancient philosopher Heraclitus the Obscure said (in one of his less obscure moments): 'Nothing is permanent but change.' And change is good if it puts you back in control of your life. One way of relieving work-related stress is to look at re-tooling yourself. New skills may make your current job easier to cope with; they can also assist you in finding a completely new job, perhaps in an unrelated field.

If you have no intention of leaving your present job but feel that the cause of your stress is lack of appropriate skills to do the job properly, the sensible option in the first instance is to talk either to your manager or personnel officer about training or gaining specific qualifications. You might find your employers willing to pay either in full or in part, for your training expenses. At the very least they might consider giving you time off for study. Before approaching them with your plan, research what training you need, where you can do it, the time and costs involved, and the benefit to your employers. If nothing else, this will show them that you are really serious about your personal training needs.

Career Development Loans (CDL): Alternatively you may feel that the solution is to change your job or career and start afresh. To do so, however, you may need new skills and qualifications and acquiring these can cost money. One way of paying for training – although this does not cover a degree or post-graduate study – is by taking out a Career Development Loan. A CDL is a deferred repayment bank loan to help pay for vocational learning or education.

- You can borrow between £300 and £8,000 to help fund up to two years of learning plus (if relevant) up to one year's practical work experience if part of the course.
- The Department for Education and Skills (DfES) pays the interest on your loan while you are studying and up to one month after the course finishes.
- You then repay the loan over an agreed period at a fixed rate of interest.
- CDLs are available through three banks: Barclays, The Cooperative Bank and The Royal Bank of Scotland.
- For more information look at the web site **www.lifelonglearning.co.uk/cdl**

You don't necessarily have to leave your job while you re-train. There are countless courses from legal, management, book-keeping and administration, to personnel, catering, horticultural and plumbing, that you can do evening, weekend, part-time or by correspondence. Contact your local IAG or Learning Direct for information on these and other courses. Prices vary and you might find a course cheap enough to let you forgo a loan. Having a positive goal to work towards can be enough to alleviate some of the negative effects of work-related stress, and you may find at the same time that it re-energises your life.

Further options: down-shifting, part-time work, flexible working or early retirement.

As Dolly Parton sang in the 1980 film *Nine to Five*:

> *Nine to five, they've got you where they want you;*
> *There's a better life, and you dream about it, don't you?*[5]

Sound familiar? Literally hundreds of thousands of people in the UK dream of a better life beyond the confines of a stressful 9 to 5 job. An estimated 1.4 million people in Britain have 'downshifted', upping stakes and moving from their jobs in the city to the cleaner air – and lower-paying jobs – of the countryside; a recent survey of workers in urban areas of Wales and the West Country found 828,000 more people with dreams of joining them.[6] Many people have found down-shifting the answer to, among other things, their mid-life crises. They resigned from their high-flying jobs, sold their high-value properties in the city, and moved their families lock, stock and barrel to the countryside where they attempted to forge a living off the land or from some low-income scheme. The experience, with its ups and downs, is described by Daniel Butler and his partner Bel Crewe in their book, *Urban Dreams, Rural Realities: In Search of the Good Life,* published in 1999. Butler, a business journalist living and working in London with his partner, decided on his 30th birthday to move to the countryside and, with the proceeds from their two flats, bought a four-bed 16th century farmhouse in Wales. It wasn't long before Butler exchanged business journalism for the tranquillity of writing about rural issues. For these two down-shifters, the dream has come true.

Downshifting can mean changing to a less materialistic lifestyle, earning less and working part-time or putting together a portfolio of jobs to bring in enough money to pay the bills. For some people, the reduction in stress that downshifting brings outweighs the inconveniences, while, for others, having to watch every penny only adds to their stress levels. What type are you?

Selling your property and moving to something smaller in a cheaper area is one way to reduce costs and free up some money to support your downshifting. Follow some of the suggestions on cutting costs in the previous section on finances so you know the minimum you can live on and then you can match income earning strategies to meet your needs.

If that sounds a little too drastic other options open might be to reduce your working hours, change your work routine and work more flexibly, or simply to **retire early**. More and more people are exercising this latter option. Despite the fact that we are living longer these days, we are also quitting the workforce, according to a recent study published for the Joseph Rowntree Foundation, at a younger and younger age.[7] Decisions to retire early vary widely, but in most cases people in Britain leave the workforce prematurely because of personal motives (such as having to care for aged parents) as well as ones related to specific conditions in the work-place.[8] Unsurprisingly, one of these conditions, identified in a study of NHS nurses, is workplace stress: many nurses over the age of 50 admitted that they were taking early retirement because of high levels of stress.[9] By cruel irony, the early retirement of large numbers of nurses – 10,000 leave the NHS each year – has been pinpointed as causing an increased stress-load for those left behind, thus creating a potential snowball.

Experiences of early retirement vary, according to Sue Arthur from the National Centre for Social Research. Those workers with the least choice and control tended to experience the greatest difficulties, whereas those with stronger financial and employment circumstances experience an easier transition. However, Arthur found that people generally did not get overly het up over financial worries when they retired early, since not having the strain of working outweighed other factors, such as having a lower income.

This option may not be appropriate for those under sixty as their pension fund might be insufficient, but before ruling out the idea, take professional pension advice. If you are close to retirement age, there are schemes that will allow you to reduce working hours without affecting your final retirement package. Thus you could work part-time for a year or two before retiring, which could help alleviate work-related stress without affecting your pension at retirement. If retirement is not a realistic option at this stage of your life then perhaps **part-time working** may be an answer, especially as researchers have found that full-time employment is linked to greater stress than part-time work. A poll carried out for Channel 4 by Taylor Nelson Sofres Phonebus found that out of 534 adults in full and part-time work, only 29% of part-time workers reported feeling stressed as opposed to 45% of full-timers.[10] So why not try part-time work for a couple of years while you give your body time to recover from prolonged stress? Once well enough, you can revert to full-time work if you want or need to. After all, there will be plenty of time for you to work in the future. Already in many European countries, such as Sweden and Germany, the official retirement age is 70, and the falling birth rate in Europe means, experts predict, that this could be raised in future another five years to 75. It is unlikely that Britain alone will keep the retirement age at 65 for long. Therefore, a year or two working part-time should not affect your right to work or your pension fund, as there will be – for better or worse – plenty of time to catch up.

Alternatively, why not consider a **portfolio of careers** where you make up an income from several different jobs or employers? This may not suit everyone as it will probably mean taking responsibility for your own NI contributions, tax and pension payments. Unless you are someone who does not fluster easily, you could find that the insecurity of juggling different commitments actually adds to your stress levels.

Or what about **flexible working?** Since 2004, as we have seen in an earlier chapter, the law has been helping parents or carers of elderly relatives by offering new working conditions, to enable them to meet their home as well as work commitments. But if you are 'child-free' and don't have a parent at home, it is good to know that there are some enlightened companies out there who are committed to flexible working for all staff. Here are some suggestions that, put to your boss, could make flexible working a reality; but remember some jobs by their very nature are unsuited to flexible working, and your employer has the right to refuse your request whatever your circumstances. If you are a receptionist and part of your job is to meet and greet the public, yet you want to work from home – well, think again! However, you'll never know if you don't ask, and this is the first step towards regaining some control over your stressed life.

- Be realistic before approaching your employer. Ensure that your role is capable of becoming more flexible.
- Give your employer clear reasons why you want to work more flexibly. You might be surprised how understanding he/she can be.
- Write a thorough plan of when and how the change could take effect.
- Anticipate any objections your employer might raise and have solutions at the ready. If you are asking to work more from home, point out that the latest IT equipment means you are never far from communication links.
- List all the advantages of your proposal for both you and your employer. Back this up with reports and statistics on the negative effects of work-related stress and give positive examples of companies that are open to flexible working for all. You can find this information on the Department of Trade and Industry's Work-Life Balance web pages.
- Offer to have a trial run for several months with a review date planned. Agree from the outset that you are prepared to work with your employer in finding ways of making flexible working benefit you both.
- Give your employer time to mull over your suggestions but make a future date to discuss them further.
- If your employer will not give a valid reason for refusing to consider your proposals, then maybe it is time to consider looking for a new job that will accommodate your needs.

Taking a sabbatical

Richard Morrison, a columnist in *The Times,* has lamented that the average eighteen year-old thinks it is his or her right to take a gap year before university to get over the stress of A'levels. This inalienable right usually includes travelling to the other side of world, seeing wonderful sights, and lazing on a beach. Green with envy, Morrison asks: 'Why do *they* need a gap year? If anyone does, it's us: the frazzled middle-agers whose sole remaining functions in life seem to be financing our children's pleasures, tending our ailing parents and paying our eternal mortgages.'[11] This dire description may not hold for every 'middle-ager', but Morrison does have a point. No-one wants to stop young adults taking time out to travel and widen their horizons, but why should it be their exclusive privilege when statistics show that so many people in the UK are suffering from work-related stress and could likewise do with a break?

One solution to alleviating work-related stress is to allow employees to get on and off the treadmill by offering sabbaticals. To make this a feasible option, mortgage and pension packages would need to be amended to allow for gaps in payments. In recent years Britain has adopted a 'work-till-you-drop' ethos, whereas our cousins in Australia still allow employees the opportunity to take time out – either paid or unpaid – to recharge their batteries. The Australian Long Service Act of 1955 entitles employees to take three months paid leave after 15 years continuous service. And although it has its origins back in the late 1860's, when employees of the Crown were permitted to take into account the sailing time for a return trip to England, long service leave has been preserved and is deeply appreciated by many Australians. And continuous service these days means all periods of employment, whether broken or continuous, combined to determine the years of service.

At present there is no UK or EU legislation dealing directly with sabbaticals, but more British companies are recognising that their employees desire a chance to take time out and re-charge. Companies such as the John Lewis Partnership allow employees to take 26 weeks paid leave after 26 years of service, whilst the *Guardian* newspaper allows four weeks paid leave in addition to annual leave after employees complete four years of service. The trend is for companies to introduce policies that offer up to one week's sabbatical leave for each completed year of service beyond a fixed period of time.

Morrison argues that there is a 'massive dissatisfaction with the way we organise (or *don't* organise) the pattern of work, play, study and family responsibilities throughout our lives. This,' he says, 'is a dam waiting to burst. The only question is when and how.'[12] If you are one of those dissatisfied with your working life and are interested in taking a sabbatical, why not talk to your employer and at least see if it is possible? Provided that cover can be found for your position, there are certainly some employers who would consider your request and regard it as beneficial to the company as well as you – because a happy worker is a productive worker.

Becoming your own boss

Sally, a physiotherapist from Bristol, was bullied by her manager and, after several months off on sick leave to recuperate, decided to leave her job and start her own business. Since making her decision, Sally has not looked back but admits that she would not have had the courage to take this step had her job not become so miserable. Running your own business is not in itself free from worries or stress, but as long as you do your research extensively before making the leap, it can be the chance to realise a long-held dream.

If you have no experience of running your own business, you would be well advised to get some professional advice before taking the leap. Wherever you are situated in the UK, there will be advice centres such as Business Link, offering a free 'first stop signposting' service that will direct you to local business support organisations. One activity worth considering is a one-day course from Business Link that costs around £10 (free for the unemployed) and details everything involved in starting up your own business. It highlights the reasons why businesses fail, the importance of market research, the legal requirements involved, financial considerations, and how to plan for the long-term future. A lot to cover in one day – and more than enough to scare away the half-hearted!

Whole books are written on the topic of starting your own business. This section is intended merely to give a few pointers to whet your appetite and not to act as a comprehensive guide. However, one of your first steps in setting up your own business is to write a business plan that will focus your ideas. This is also essential if you intend to request a 'start-up loan'.

For a business plan to be effective, you will need to undertake market research. For example, what is your product, what is your target market, what is the competition, and what are your costs?

Next you must decide how you should operate under the law. You can become a **Sole Trader.** This means that if your business fails – worst case scenario – you will be personally liable for any debts. As a self-employed worker, you do not need to register the business, but you will need to notify the Inland Revenue for tax and National Insurance purposes. As a Sole Trader you will also need to keep full records of your business and personal finances, and to submit an annual Self Assessment tax return. Some people find these tasks in themselves extremely stressful, but there is always help at hand at your local Tax Office, or you can find an accountant who specialises in small businesses.

Limited Companies, by contrast, are legal entities in their own right. Taxation for them is treated differently than for Sole Traders, as the profits of the company are subject to corporation tax. The directors of a company are employees and must pay income tax and NI at source through the PAYE system. **Partnerships** consist of between two and twenty people choosing to trade together as a business, each partner being responsible for the partnership's debts.

There are so many things to consider when starting up your own business. Should you work from home or rent space? Do you need special licences or insurances to trade? Have you considered fire safety, and health and safety regulations? Are you clear about legal requirements under the Data Protection Act if you store names and addresses? Will you need to take on any employees? Will you be liable for VAT? A business adviser can help you fine-tune your business plan and make sure you do not forget any important details. Visit your nearest Business Link for local contacts.

Sally did just that, speaking to a business adviser when she decided to set up her own private physiotherapy practice. While healing, she had come to the conclusion that she could no longer continue in her present employment. She wanted a less stressful job where she was more in control of her life and career, even if meant earning less. This last point was a major step forward for Sally, as she had remained for too long in her previous job because she felt she needed the money.

Her business idea was to specialise in after-surgery physiotherapy, concentrating on hip and knee replacements and fractures. After attending an hour's informal chat, she signed up for the one-day course that Business Link offered on 'Setting up Your Own Business'. Armed with basic information and a template for a Business Plan, she set to work researching the feasibility of her ideas.

Before Sally started seriously on her business plan, however, she sat down with her husband and worked out their monthly outgoings. She was fortunate that her husband was a high earner in a job he enjoyed and was able to cover the mortgage on his own if necessary. Even so, they worked out a plan where they could cut back on non-essentials until Sally was more financially secure.

Sally then set to work on her business plan. She checked out the competition in her area and found, to her delight, that there was a gap in the market for her specialisation. She then researched the best places to advertise her services, including local GP surgeries, hospitals, the internet, local advertising magazines, residential homes for the elderly, the University of the Third Age, and a physiotherapy web site. Deciding to network, she also listed all the professional contacts she had made when working as a state-registered physiotherapist.

Sally decided that before she registered as a Sole Trader, however, she would find part-time work for several months as a locum physiotherapist. She knew this would not be well paid but it would ease her back into work, allowing her slowly to regain her confidence. Whilst doing locum work she left her business card where appropriate, and as a result she was offered a room to rent in a local GP surgery where she could practice two days a week, including the use of the surgery receptionists to book her appointments.

Before she could start practicing, Sally had to find the money to buy some equipment, to keep up her professional registration with the Chartered Society of Physiotherapy, to take out appropriate insurances, and of course to pay the rent for her business premises. Her business adviser went through the options with her, and she decided to ask for a business start-up loan from one of the High Street banks to top up £3,000 of her own savings. After about five months of locum work and several appointments with her business adviser, Sally was finally ready to start trading. 'I'm still only part-time', she says, 'but I am now working three days a week instead of two. The pace of life really suits me, and I actually have more time to enjoy my home life. Being bullied was an absolutely terrible experience, but at least I've manage to make some good come of it all'.

It's sometimes said that finding a full-time job – drafting your CV, scouring the job adverts, filling in applications, going to interviews – is a full-time job in itself. Down-shifting, setting up your own business, or working out plans for flexible working, sabbaticals or early retirement can likewise become full-time jobs. But, as we have seen, if you do your homework properly, the rewards of liberating yourself from the cause of your stress can be immense.

6 COPING STRATEGIES

As we have seen, work-related stress can cause all sorts of physical, emotional and behavioural reactions. It should therefore be taken seriously to prevent permanent damage to your health. This section is not about cure – the source of the stress has to be identified for that – but rather about the coping strategies that can assist healing: medications, therapies, and mechanisms for regaining control of your life. It is designed to give you an idea of what kind of help is available; it is up to you to experiment with different approaches in order to find the method that suits you. Any healing should be a holistic experience, which means you must discover the source of your dis-ease before looking for its cure. Many people mix traditional healing methods with alternative remedies; unless you are taking oral medicine, nearly all are compatible. Remember: coping strategies learnt now can prevent a recurrence of stress in the future.

Doctors and Pills

When Aldous Huxley published *Brave New World* in 1932 he introduced to his readers a hypothetical drug called Soma. The wonder drug of the twenty-fifth century, Soma would lift the mood and rid the mind of any negative thoughts. It was, in essence, a drug that prevented depression. Little could Huxley know that six decades later, in the years 1992/93, spending by the National Health Service (NHS) on psychiatric drugs similar to Soma would amount to £159 million, or 5.2% of the entire NHS budget for that year.[1] Indeed, so widespread is the use of antidepressants in Western medicine that we are literally excreting them into the ecosystem: a study by the University of Texas has found traces of Prozac – probably the best-known of the antidepressants – in river water and fish.[2]

According to Department of Health figures, around 20% of women and 14% of men in England suffer from depression at any one time; the Mental Health Foundation claims the figures are in fact higher, affecting one in four adults in the UK.[3] As we have seen in Chapter Two, work-related stress can cause depression because the stress hormone cortisol, if released in excess, can inhibit the production of serotonin, a chemical that affects our mood. That is why doctors will often prescribe anti-depressants called Selective Serotonin Re-uptake Inhibitors (SSRIs) for depression caused by work-related stress. The aim of SSRIs is to influence positively the serotonin in the brain. Besides Fluozotine (Prozac), the most common drugs in this group are:

- Sertraline (Soloft)
- Paroxetine (Paxil)
- Fluvoxamine (Luvox)
- Citalopram (Celexa)
- Escitalopra (Lexapro)

For severe cases of depression, or in cases where SSRIs do not work, the Tricyclic Antidepressants (TCAs) are prescribed. These are an older type of antidepressant which tend to have more side effects. The most common in this group are:

- Amitriptyline (Elavil)
- Clomipramine (Anafranil)
- Desipramine (Norpramin)
- Doxepin (Adapin)
- Imipramine (Tofranil)
- Nortriptyline (Pamelor)
- Protriptyline (Vivactil)
- Trimipramine (Surmontil)

There is a further group of antidepressants called Monoamine Oxidase Inhibitors (MAOIs). These are less common and are often used to treat elderly people, as their side effects are relatively mild. However, you cannot mix MAOIs with other drugs because of possible negative reactions. Common MAOIs are:

- Phenelzine (Nardil)
- Tranylcypromine (Parnate)

Finally, there are Atypical Antidepressants. These are chemically distinct from SSRIs in that they balance serotonin and norepinephrine levels. (Norepinephrine is a neurotransmitter that works in the sympathetic nervous system and is released into the bloodstream in response to short-term stress.) The SSRIs, on the other hand, maintain levels of the excitatory neurohormone serotonin in the brain, but do not alter levels of norepinephrine. Atypical antidepressants are often prescribed when SSRIs have not worked. Included among them are:

- Bupropion (Wellburin)
- Mirtazapine (Remeron)
- Nefazodone (Serzone)
- Trazadone (Desyrel)

More than two thirds of people who take antidepressants get better, but, like any drug, they can cause side effects, and in extreme cases they can even increase depression. For this reason, your doctor will regularly monitor your progress in the first few months. Side effects will vary from drug to drug, but common ones are:

- dry mouth
- sexual problems
- nausea
- tremor
- insomnia
- blurred vision
- constipation
- dizziness

Antidepressants can typically take 3 – 5 weeks to start working and sometimes they simply don't suit. Joy, a bank teller, was prescribed an antidepressant and found it really didn't help her at all. 'Maybe I wasn't on it long enough, but I stopped taking it after about a month. What helped me enormously through my crisis was sleep, and I didn't seem to need much help with that.' And yet, Mark, a deputy retail manager, reluctantly accepted a prescription for Prozac after months of being bullied by his manager. 'It took a few weeks for it to kick in, but when it did I just felt calmer and I suddenly realised that I wasn't festering for days on end over things that were said.' Mark was also prescribed Trazadone, which he took for a couple of months Trazadone, a non-addictive tranquilliser that does not interfere with Prozac, helped Mark to sleep at night.

With so many antidepressants on the market, how does your doctor know which is right for you? Unfortunately, some guess-work and experimentation is usually involved. According to Dr. Andrew A. Nierenberg, associate director of the depression clinical and research programme at the General Hospital in Boston, matching patients to antidepressants is opinion-based, not data-based.[4] One of the problems with antidepressant drugs is that, because of the variation in the structure and makeup of receptors in the cell membranes of each individual, they will only work for about 85% of patients. As there is no concrete data on what will work on whom, doctors have to make subjective judgements. As studies have shown that there is no difference in effectiveness between SSRIs and the older TCAs for treating mild to moderate depression,[5] some doctors make decisions based on the cost factor – TCAs are cheaper. Indeed, it was predicted in 1993 that if 70% of TCAs in the UK were replaced by the more expensive SSRIs, the total annual cost of antidepressants in general practice would rise from £88 million to £200 million a year.[6]

Antidepressants will not solve your problems for you, but they may give you a break from the exhausting cycle of worry and fretfulness that depression can cause, and that in turn can allow you to begin to address the problems – a bullying manager or an unmanageable workload – underlying your depression. They may also protect the brain from the damage which depression causes to the hippocampus – the area of the brain involved in learning and memory. These days, antidepressants are non-addictive, but patients must withdraw from them slowly to avoid sudden side effects. Antidepressants will suit some people and not others; always discuss any concerns with your doctor, who will work with you to find a drug that suits you and your particular circumstances.

Cognitive (Behavioural) Therapy: Accentuating the positive

Imagine you are walking along the pavement when you see your friend coming from the opposite direction on the other side of a busy street. You wave to him, but he fails to respond. How does this make you feel? And what assumption do you make about his behaviour? If you think your friend is deliberately ignoring you, you may feel angry, confused or sad. On the other hand, you may decide your friend did not see you, in which case you will not be upset at all.

What is it? Cognitive therapy concentrates on the connections between how we think, how we feel and how we behave. It trains the mind to respond in a positive way to what may be perceived as negative events. People who successfully use this technique – whether subconsciously or consciously – are those who learn to see the wine glass as being half full, as opposed to being half empty!

The difference between cognitive therapy and counselling is that the cognitive therapist takes an active part in solving the problem. He or she will not simply nod wisely and expect you to find the answers on your own. Rather, it is a structured and focused therapy with identifiable agreed goals. A cognitive therapist can be a clinical psychologist, psychiatrist or nurse therapist, and your GP should be able to recommend one in your area. For more information refer to the British Association for Behavioural and Cognitive Psychotherapies, see **www.babcp.org.uk**.

Is this a new therapy? Yes and no. In *Mourning and Melancholia*, Sigmund Freud wrote, as early as 1917, that melancholy (depression) can occur in response to an imaginary or perceived loss, and that our self-criticisms – automatic negative thoughts about ourselves – are responsible in part for depression. But it was Dr. Aaron Beck, an American psychologist born in 1921, who, after years of research, founded cognitive therapy in the 1970s. It wasn't until this period that psychologists started to recognise the effectiveness of cognitive therapy in healing many aspects of depression. Beck's methods became so popular that in 1999 he founded the Academy of Cognitive Therapy, which is based at the University of Pennsylvania, where research on the subject continues today.

What can it treat? According to the New York Institute for Cognitive and Behavioural Therapies, cognitive therapy can treat the following conditions, many of which are caused, directly or indirectly, by stress at work:[7]

- Depression and mood swings
- Shyness and social anxiety
- Panic attacks and phobias
- Obsessions and compulsions
- Chronic anxiety or worry
- Post-traumatic stress symptoms
- Insomnia and other sleep problems
- Job, career or school difficulties
- Feeling 'stressed out'
- Low self-esteem
- Inadequate coping skills, or ill-chosen methods of coping
- Passivity, procrastination and 'passive aggression'
- Difficulty in keeping feelings within bounds

What can I expect? This depends on the individual, but most courses of cognitive therapy last from 8–12 weeks, based on one 50-minute session a week. Clients are given homework and tasks to complete, such as keeping diaries of their thoughts and reactions to stressful events. These reactions will then be discussed with the therapist during the session. Analysing stressful events and our response to them, cognitive therapists claim, help us to learn new ways of looking at the problem. The mind is trained, that is, to avoid the dark and thorny path of negativity, paranoia and self-criticism that leads to the dead-end of anxiety and depression, in favour of the high road of optimistic coping and realistic self-management. So even if it transpires that your friend was deliberately ignoring you, this slight will not start a sort of mental landslide of self-doubt and self-criticism that spreads into other aspects of your life. You cannot change other people's thoughts and behaviour – but you can change your own!

Anger Management: Taking a deep breath

A common symptom of stress is anger: anger because you have too much work; anger because you are about to be made redundant; anger because your boss is working against you instead of with you … there are so many things that can infuriate us at work. Feeling angry is a completely normal and often a healthy emotion. However, if this rage spins out of control, it can not only affect our overall quality of life but, as we have seen in Chapter Two, cause serious health problems such as high blood pressure, strokes and heart attacks. Anger, therefore, like a negative thought, is something that must be managed.

What is anger? Anger is an emotional state that is accompanied, like other emotions, by physiological and biological changes. When you get angry, your heart rate and blood pressure rise, as do your energy hormones, epinephrine (more commonly known as adrenaline) and noradrenaline. Like fear, anger is an instinctive way of responding to a threat. However, in modern society it is unacceptable for us physically to lash out at anyone or any thing that annoys us, so we have adopted conscious and unconscious ways, both overt and covert, of dealing with the emotion. Anger can be expressed out loud by cursing, fighting and throwing things, or it can be expressed quietly, by withdrawing socially, sulking or becoming ill.

Are some people naturally angrier than others? The American psychologist, Dr Jerry Deffenbacher, professor of psychology at Colorado State University, an expert on anger, thinks that some people are just more hot-headed than others.[8] This could be due to their genetic or physiological make-up, or it could be socio-cultural, for example, if they have not been taught how to deal with angry feelings in a constructive way. Research has also found that many angry people come from disruptive and chaotic families with communication difficulties. Whatever the case, however, everyone can be taught to manage their anger. The cost of not doing so – in terms of both physical and mental health – is simply too high.

Anger strategies

As Aristotle wrote, 'Anyone can become angry – that is easy. But to be angry with the right person, to the right degree, at the right time, for the right purpose, and in the right way; this is not easy.' That is why learning strategies to keep anger at bay, or to use it productively, are essential.

Relaxation techniques: When you find yourself in a tense situation, follow some of these simple steps to help calm you down.

- Take deep breaths, breathing deeply right from your diaphragm.
- Repeat to yourself while taking deep breaths a word or phrase such as 'calm down' or 'relax'. Do this as many times as you feel necessary.
- Visualize a relaxing scene or situation from your memory or imagination.

Cognitive Restructuring: Cognitive therapy, covered in the previous section, can also be a useful tool in changing the way you think about what makes you angry. Be careful about the words you express when angry. Words like 'never' or 'always' allow no way out of a problem. For example, saying to someone 'you *never* do it properly' or 'you *always* make mistakes' backs that person into a corner. Keep reminding yourself that getting angry is a waste of energy and won't solve the problem; you need calm energy in order to find a solution to whatever has made you angry.

Humour: Learning not to take yourself too seriously is important in anger management. Humour can be used to help you look at situations differently. You can always take David Brent's advice from the popular BBC sitcom, *The Office:* 'If your boss is getting you down, look at him through the prongs of a fork and imagine him in jail.' It won't necessarily solve anything but it should bring a smile to your face! However, be careful not to hide the problem by pretending you are not angry when really you are, because bottling up your anger is not the answer either. Too often this will cause resentment to build up. Use humour to face the cause of your anger constructively. But remember, too, that sarcastic humour is just another expression of anger.

Communication: Angry people tend to jump to conclusions and then act on them immediately. So when you feel angry, slow down and take stock. Don't say the first thing that comes in to your head; listen to what is being said, and think before you reply. If you need some space, remove yourself from the scene. Always try to keep communication lines open.

Problem solving: Not all anger is misplaced, but not all problems can be solved in the way you want. Try not to focus on finding a solution; rather, focus on ways of handling the situation. You may find the solution comes in its own time.

For more information on anger management treatments refer to the British Association of Anger Management at **www.angermanage.co.uk.**

Assertiveness Training: Standing up for your rights

Which is better, asks Hamlet in Act 3 of William Shakespeare's famous play: to suffer the 'slings and arrows of outrageous fortune', or to 'take arms against a sea of troubles, / And by opposing, end them'?[9] To suffer passively or to fight – a dilemma familiar to many who suffer from work-related stress. Is it better to accept unhappiness at work, or should you stand up for your rights, irrespective of the consequences? That is indeed the question!

Work-related stress can prompt a host of feelings ranging from passivity and self-deprecation to fear and anger. These emotions often go hand in hand with an inability to express ourselves appropriately. For example, you might wish to say to your boss, 'I have so much work that I am having to stay late every night to finish it. Not only does this make me feel tired the next day, but it is also affecting my family life'. Instead you may give the impression that you do not mind – although, deep down, you do. Of course, unassertive people are not always passive and accepting; sometimes they react with inappropriate and unproductive aggression. An aggressive response in the case above might be to blow your top and complain loudly to your boss at the unfairness of it all. This sort of reaction prevents a compromise, and may cause your boss to react by likewise becoming angry. If only you could make yourself understood without ruffling anyone's feathers ... Well, with a little help, you can!

What does assertiveness mean? Being assertive is the ability to express yourself and your rights without violating the rights of others. When being assertive you can have direct, open and honest communication that allows you to feel self-confident and in control of everyday situations.

Believing in your rights: Despite the mistaken assumption that it is selfish to put your needs before others, you are doing more harm than good by failing to be assertive. For example:

- In allowing yourself to be dominated, you lose your self-respect.
- In concealing your true feelings, you become dishonest.
- In being submissive, you lose the respect of others.
- In allowing yourself to be a doormat, you are oppressed.
- In failing to express yourself honestly, you may resort to subtle manipulation, thereby creating resentment.
- In complying when you disagree, you reward your oppressor.

However, stating your needs aggressively can also have negative results. For example:

- In acting aggressively, you can humiliate and anger others.
- In acting aggressively, you can lose the respect of others.

If assertiveness means the ability to express your thoughts and feelings in a way that clearly states your needs, as Regina Ryan and John Travis argue in *The Wellness Workbook*,[10] you must believe you have a legitimate right to have those needs. Unassertive people often forget their basic rights, which are:

- The right to pursue your own goals and dreams and to decide how to lead your life.
- The right not to justify or explain your actions or feelings.
- The right to have your own values, beliefs, opinions and emotions.
- The right to tell others how you wish to be treated.
- The right to say 'No', 'I don't know' or 'I don't understand'.

- The right to change your mind.
- The right to ask for information or help.
- The right to have positive relationships that allow you to feel comfortable and free to express yourself honestly.
- The right to be alone even if others would prefer your company.
- The right to change or end relationships if they do not meet your needs.

Techniques for assertiveness: By believing in your basic rights and learning to say what you mean in the correct way, you are on the right track for meeting your personal needs. So:

- Be specific and use precise statements to say what you want, think or feel.
- Use statements such as 'Would you …?' 'I want to …' 'I don't want you to …' 'I have a different opinion. I think that …' or 'I liked it when you did that.'
- Deliver your message directly. If you want to say something to June, tell June; do not tell everyone *except* June.
- Own your statements. Make statements using 'I'. For example 'I don't agree with you' rather than, 'you are wrong'.
- Ask for feedback. Encourage people to be clear in what they want. For example, 'Am I being clear?', 'What would you like me to do?' or 'How do you see the situation?'
- Remember that you also communicate non-verbally with voice tone, eye contact, facial expression, gesture and posture, and these can have an effect on others.

Being assertive does not guarantee you fair treatment. It does not mean that others will be assertive rather than aggressive in return, and it certainly does not mean you will always get what you want. It will, however, give you self-respect in your dealings with co-workers and pride in the knowledge that you are asking for your needs to be met in a non-aggressive, non-threatening manner. Who knows? If Hamlet had received assertiveness training, his story may have had a completely different outcome!

Life Coaching: Help from the touchline

Positive thinking and affirmations are all very well for the determined, but what if you need the encouragement and support of someone else to chivvy you along with your ideas on how to change your life and relieve stress? If this sounds like you, then maybe a life coach can help.

Life coaching, like cognitive therapy, is an interactive process that helps you to develop more rapidly and produce the results that you want. A professional coach will customize a programme to suit your needs and will provide feedback to help you along. At the end of the day, however, you are the one who must assume responsibility for taking action.

Coaching is different from counselling, as it does not focus on removing psychological pain or emotional disorders. What it *can* cover is:

- Career transition
- Career planning
- Career decisions
- Budgeting and financial planning
- Organization
- Creativity
- Life vision and enhancement
- Life planning

What to expect from a coach: You will have a personal interview either face-to-face or by telephone and desired outcomes and priorities for action will be identified. In subsequent sessions you may be asked to complete certain actions that will help you to reach your goals. Assessments are sometimes used to support the process and provide objective information to enhance the individual's self-awareness. Coaching is an individual process and can take between 3 – 6 months.

Tips:
When choosing a coach it is advisable to:

- Research coaching on the internet so you are clear what is on offer.
- Understand your objectives. A coach can only help you to achieve them if you know what they are!
- Interview several coaches before deciding. Check out qualifications and experience. Ask for references. In the first instance refer to the web site **www.coaching-life.co.uk**
- When choosing a coach, look for specialized skills they might that suit your needs. For example, if your goal is to change your job, have they experience with career transition clients?
- There should be a connection between you and the coach for it to work. Make sure the relationship feels right.
- Ensure you complete all the tasks the coach asks of you.

Managing Panic Attacks and Hyperventilation

As we saw in Chapter Two, Fay experienced a particularly frightening panic attack in the supermarket, brought on by stress, and she found that these attacks occurred regularly when her annual short-term contract came up for renewal. Many people suffering from stress, work-related or otherwise, experience panic attacks and hyperventilation. These frightening episodes are the way the body reacts to a fearful or stressful situation. If you suffer any of the following symptoms, you may be prone to hyperventilation which can lead to a full-blown panic attack:

- Are you often short of breath?
- Do you sometimes feel as if you are suffocating?
- Do you yawn, sigh or take big gulps of air?
- Do you hold your breath or take very quick breaths when frightened?
- Do you experience chest pain, or sensations of tingling, prickling or numbness?

If you suffer from any of the above symptoms, you may be breathing incorrectly. Count how many breaths you take in one minute. The average should be 10-12.

Slow down your breathing: To reduce symptoms of hyperventilation, carbon dioxide must be increased, but steadied, in the blood stream. The most tried and trusted way is to blow in to a paper bag. However, this is useful only during an attack – and you must have a bag handy!

The following breathing exercise works as a preventative and should be practiced four times a day, or at the first sign of panic or anxiety:

- Breathe normally, then hold your breath and count to 5.
- When you reach 5, breathe out and say the word 'relax'.
- Breathe in through your nose for 3 seconds, then exhale, also through the nose, for 3 seconds.
- After one minute (10 breaths), hold your breath for 5 seconds, then repeat the above process.
- Continue until you feel calmer.

Drugs treatments: Panic attacks are a serious condition, and sometimes the patient will be prescribed medication to combat them. The antidepressants Paroxetine (Paxil) and Sertraline (Zoloft) are effective in preventing anxiety and panic attacks. Other drugs such as Alprazolam (Xanax) and Clonazepam (Klonopin) give relief from fear and anxiety but should be taken only for a few weeks to a few months. Always seek advice from your doctor.

Drug free treatments: In addition to drugs, certain therapies have proven effective in treating panic attacks. Psychotherapy, Cognitive (behavioural) therapy and Hypnotherapy have all been successful in getting to the cause of panic attacks and finding new ways of dealing with them. Tai chi and Qi Kung are martial arts that use slow movements to stretch and relax the body. The Alexander Technique releases the muscle tension that causes aching neck and shoulders and can cause restricted breathing due to tension in the chest. Meditation relaxes the mind and Bach Flower Remedies, available from your local chemist, can help with feelings of anxiety. The Linden Method, created by Charles Linden, uses techniques that tackle all aspects of anxiety by breaking them down, addressing them and 'disempowering' them.

Fay took six months to get well after work-related stress caused her physical and mental exhaustion. During her healing process she took up Tai Chi. 'At first it was hard to concentrate because the movements were so slow,' she explains. 'But now I really miss it if I don't practice once a day. The bit I found the hardest – breathing slowly whilst concentrating on each movement – is the bit that I now find the most relaxing.'

Bagging Some Zeds: Easing insomnia

A flock of sheep that leisurely pass by
One after one; the sound of rain, and bees
Murmuring; the fall of rivers, winds and seas,
Smooth fields, white sheets of water, and pure sky –
I've thought of all by turns, and still I lie
Sleepless …

William Wordsworth (1780–1850), 'To Sleep'

How many times have you, like Wordsworth, lain awake counting sheep? Insomnia is, of course, a common symptom of stress. The more difficulties Mark, a deputy retail manager, encountered at work, the less he could sleep. 'I tried counting sheep, using imagery to relax my body and even bought some over-the-counter sleeping medicine,' he explained. 'Nothing worked because I could not stop thinking about work or my manager and the less sleep I got, the more mistakes I was making at work.'

Some people can get by with only 6 hours sleep whilst others need 10 hours a night – there is no standard for all. Whatever your personal requirements, too little can cause depression, irritability and the inability to function efficiently. Work-related stress can cause insomnia (see Chapter Two), and insomniacs the world over can empathise with the American writer F. Scott Fitzgerald's lament that 'the worst thing in the world is to try to sleep and not to'. So, what can be done?

What are the effects of insomnia? The popular television serial *Star Trek: The Next Generation* covered the effects of sleep deprivation in an episode called 'Night Terrors', first broadcast in 1991. The crew of the USS *Enterprise* were caught in a spatial anomaly that prevented them from reaching REM sleep, and as a consequence many of them suffered paranoid delusions and hallucinations, and became unable to function properly.

The 'spatial anomaly' may have been science fiction, but the depiction of the results of insomnia was real enough. The function of sleep is to rest and repair the body. We dream when we are in a deep sleep, and dreaming has certain psychological benefits. The state of deep sleep is known as Rapid Eye Movement (REM) because our eyes can be seen to flicker as they watch our dreamscape. Lack of sufficient REM sleep – as the *Enterprise* crew discovered – can lead to mood swings and affect the part of the brain that improves memory and learning. Insomnia can include the following symptoms: difficulty in falling asleep, waking too early in the morning, waking during the night and having trouble getting back to sleep, and waking up feeling unrefreshed.

Treatment

Drugs: Sleeping tablets can be prescribed for a limited period for chronic (long-term) insomnia. These work on the brain by reducing the level of mental activity, thus encouraging sleep. However, the nature of sleep will be affected and despite the fact that you may sleep longer your REM sleep (dream state) will not be so good. Moreover, some medication can cause grogginess or drowsiness, and long-term use can be addictive.

The most common sleeping tablets are benzodiasepines and include temazepam, nitrazepam, flurazepam, loprazolam and lormetzepam. Barbiturates are rarely used these days. Other sleeping tablets include chloral hydrate, chlomethiazole, zlopidem and zopiclone. Zlopidem and zopiclone are the newer drugs on the market and are designed to help sleep follow a more natural pattern. Always discuss the options with your doctor.

Drug free: L-tryptophan, found in dairy products, eggs, chicken, cashews and pumpkin seeds, is one of the essential amino acids that the body uses to make neurotransmitters such as serotonin. Serotonin helps your brain shut down for the night and then be fully awake the following day. More L-tryptophan reaches the brain if it is mixed with carbohydrates, which is why a whole-grain biscuit or sandwich can make a good night-time snack. Indeed, eating a lettuce sandwich about an hour before bed is particularly beneficial, as lettuce contains opiate-like chemicals and is sleep-inducing when mixed with the carbohydrates in wholemeal bread.[11]

Drinking a warm glass of milk before bed really *does* help you to sleep, just as your grandmother may have told you. Milk not only has L-tryptophan but calcium as well, a natural calming agent. Alternatively, a banana shake – milk and banana liquidized together – is another way to ingest L-tryptophan in order to induce sleep.

If you are a tea addict, try switching from black tea, with its caffeine that keeps you awake, to herbal teas such as chamomile, lemon verbena, lemon balm, passion flower and peppermint. They are reputed to have qualities that calm and soothe, helping you to fall asleep. The herb valerian (see Chapter 8) is a non-addictive remedy that is also known to aid sleep; a few drops of lavender oil on the pillow at night can likewise help (see Chapter 6). Cognitive therapy can also be of assistance to people having prolonged and persistent insomnia.

Tips for a good night's sleep

- Make your bedroom an inviting place with soothing colours and pleasing décor.
- Use the bedroom for sleep and sex only.
- Go to bed at the same time each night and get up at a regular time.
- Follow a routine at bedtime to relax and unwind – take a relaxing bath, listen to soothing music or read something light.
- Exercise daily but not just before bedtime.
- Make sure you have the right mattress – up-grade if it is old, lumpy or uncomfortable.
- Make sure your room is well ventilated when you sleep.
- If you wake in the night with your mind going over things, make a list of worries or actions because, as Charlotte Bronte wrote, 'a ruffled mind makes a restless pillow'.

What to avoid

- Do not watch TV in bed.
- Do not take the work to bed and never use a laptop whilst in bed.
- Do not eat in bed.
- Do not nap in the day.
- Do not consume caffeinated drinks – hot chocolate, coffee, tea or fizzy drinks - after 4pm. Caffeine works as a stimulant and will keep you awake.
- Do not drink alcohol 2-3 hours before bed.
- Do not smoke in the evening. Nicotine can cause insomnia.
- Do not eat a heavy meal in the evening, but do not go to bed hungry either, as this leads to low levels of blood sugar that can cause irritability and tiredness when you wake.
- Do not go on the Atkins diet if you suffer from insomnia. The diet forbids complex carbohydrates such as pasta, beans, brown rice and wholemeal bread; however, these foods trigger the release of serotonin which is vital for a good night's sleep.[12]

Most people suffer from insomnia sometime in their lives. Usually the phase passes without much damage apart from a few bleary-eyed days. However, work-related stress can cause unrelenting insomnia as your body permanently creates the hormone cortisol in readiness for the 'fight or flight' reaction. Tiredness can not only cause depression; it can also affect your ability to perform properly at work. That is why it is vital to get to the cause of the stress. Otherwise, all the remedies, strategies, therapies and techniques mentioned so far will do little to help, other than to cover over a deep-rooted problem. For more information on insomnia and cures, refer to the British Sleep Foundation web site **www.britishsleepfoundation.org.uk** or the Sleep Assessment Advisory Service web site **www.neuronic.com.**

Sufferers from work-related stress will not necessarily need to use all the coping strategies recommended in this chapter, but once you have your anger under control, for example, or your sleep restored, you will be ready to start feeling good about yourself again. The next chapter introduces the stressed-out worker to a selection of 'feel good' remedies and strategies. Pick one or try them all as now is the time to spend energy on *yourself* – and what is amazing is that there is no need to feel guilty, as numerous medical studies show that the body requires pampering for it to achieve its true potential.

7 THE FEEL GOOD FACTOR

It is astonishing how many people feel guilty about spending time and money on relaxation - apart from, of course, the things that are bad for us, such as booze and fags! Healthy relaxation leads us to feel much better about ourselves, but relaxing can be difficult if our bodies have been on stress alert for a prolonged period. Relaxation may be something we need to relearn. Even Sally, a professional physiotherapist whose job is to help people relax strained muscles, was shocked at how tense and knotted her neck and shoulders had become – and also how long it took her to address the problem. 'I was unaware that the stress had built up in my own body to such an extent, until I started having regular massages,' she explained. Sally found massages so beneficial as stress-busters that she continues to have them today.

Massage is one approach to relaxing a tired mind and body, but there are many other techniques that may suit your particular lifestyle, interests and wallet. Whatever you choose, learning stress-busting techniques is the first step towards feeling better about yourself. And feeling better about yourself will equip you both mentally and physically, for dealing with stress.

Massage: The human touch

The Holy Roman Emperor Frederick II, who died in 1250, was a rare species of man. Known as 'the Wonder of the World', he spoke nine languages, wrote a treatise on falconry, went on a Crusade to the Holy Land, and got himself excommunicated (not once, but twice) by the Pope, who called him the 'blasphemous beast of the Apocalypse'.

Among Frederick's many interests was the origin of language. Curious to determine what language children would use if they were raised without hearing speech, he devised an experiment: he deprived a number of newborns of touch and speech, then awaited the results. Sadly, all of the babies died before they uttered a word, a tragedy suggesting that physical touch is absolutely essential for a child's development. In 1915, Dr Henry Dwight Chapin, a New York paediatrician, discovered that this grim experiment was accidentally being repeated in hospitals in a number of American cities. Many children under the age of two began dying in hospital despite good nutrition and sanitation. Their unexpected deaths were simply attributed to *marasmus* ('wasting away') until Dr Chapin realised that the true cause was a lack of human touch: the babies had been isolated from touch for fear of catching infections from doctors and nurses or spreading it to the other babies.[1]

Touch not only makes you feel good, therefore, but is essential for your health and survival. Lack of physical contact can lead to isolation, illness and even, in these extreme cases, death. Health professionals are now recognising the benefits of touch. Dr. Joan Borysenko, a Harvard-trained medical scientist and psychologist, argues that there is too little touch in Western medicine. 'One of the complaints heard frequently,' she says, 'is that physicians don't touch their patients any more. Touch just isn't there. Years ago massage was a big part of nursing. There was so much care, so much touch, so much goodness conveyed through massage. Now nurses for the most part are as busy as physicians. They're writing charts, dealing with insurance notes, they're doing procedures, and often there is no room for massage anymore.'[2]

Hippocrates wrote in the 5th century B.C that 'the way to health is to have a scented bath and an oiled massage each day'.[3] Studies have recently shown that Hippocrates might not have been far off the mark. Numerous scientific studies have shown the physical and psychological advantages of massage. Cancer patients at the James Cancer Hospital and Research Institute in Columbus, Ohio, reported feeling less pain and anxiety after receiving therapeutic massage.[4] Likewise, medical students at the University of New Jersey Medical School showed a significant decrease in anxiety and respiratory rates when they were massaged before taking an exam. They also showed a significant increase in white blood cells and natural killer cell activity, suggesting that massage can also benefit the immune system.[5] And according to researchers at the University of South Carolina, women who suffered the death of a child experienced fewer symptoms of depression if they received regular therapeutic massage.[6]

According to the American Massage Therapeutic Association (AMTA)[7], on a physical level therapeutic massage can:

- Relieve muscle tension and stiffness
- Reduce muscle spasms
- Provide greater joint flexibility and range of motion
- Promote deeper and easier breathing
- Improve circulation of blood and movement of lymph fluids
- Reduce blood pressure
- Help relieve tension-related headaches and effects of eye strain
- Enhance health and nourishment of skin
- Improve posture
- Strengthen immune system
- Treat musculoskeletal problems

On a mental level, therapeutic massage can:

- Help relieve mental stress

- Improve ability to monitor stress signals and respond appropriately
- Reduce levels of anxiety
- Promote a relaxed state of mental alertness
- Enhance capacity for calm thinking and creativity
- Satisfy needs for caring nurturing touch
- Foster a feeling of well-being
- Create body awareness
- Increase awareness of mind-body connection

There are five main types of massage, and all will help relieve symptoms of stress:

1) *Swedish:* A holistic treatment that addresses a person's psychological, physical and emotional well-being. It involves the kneading and manipulation of muscles, tendons and ligaments. Many practitioners use massage oil.

2) *Shiatsu:* Developed in Japan, its practitioners use thumbs and palms to apply pressure to specific points in the body. In addition, gentle stretching and synchronised breathing are encouraged. There are over 600 acupressure points that lie along fourteen meridians (energy lines), each of which represents a major organ system. The application of pressure clears these energy blockages, allowing healing to commence. Usually shiatsu is practised on the floor or mat, and patients do not need to undress.

3) *Sports massage:* Using techniques of Swedish massage as well as compression, pounding, friction and stretching, this type of massage is helpful before exercise for a stimulatory effect, or after activity to release toxins, muscle spasms and knotted tissue. It is often administered to increase flexibility.

4) *Aromatherapy massage:* This is a combination of massage with the use of diluted essential oils. These oils have specific healing and emotion-inducing properties, and the massage can therefore either be stimulating, relaxing or stress-relieving. Refer to Appendix 2 for a list of essential oils that are used for relieving some of the symptoms of stress.

5) *Reflexology:* This is a Chinese form of acupressure that works on the feet by using thumb pressure on certain points of the foot. There are ten zones or energy channels, its practitioners maintain, that run vertically through the body and correspond to precise points on either the left or right foot. For example, for a stiff neck a reflexologist might apply pressure to the big toe on your right foot. Reflexology is known to relieve pain, improve circulation and reduce stress, and you can keep your clothes on – apart, that is, from your socks!

Tips:

- Many massage therapists use oils. If you have any allergies remember to mention this.
- Before the massage begins, the practitioner will ask you for details of your medical history. This must be done to ensure the therapy is right for you and under the provisions of the Data Protection Act all information must be kept confidential.
- You can request a male or female therapist, whichever makes you feel more comfortable.
- You do not have to strip naked and can keep undergarments on if you wish. You usually are covered up by a towel during the procedure, to keep from catching chills.
- Always tell the therapist if the pressure is too soft or too hard. Everyone is different.
- Close your eyes and enjoy the experience!

When not to have a massage:

- If you have a temperature, fever, or viral infection. Infections can spread further in the body via the lymphatic system.
- If you have undergone a serious operation.
- If you have heart problems.
- If you have acute back pain.
- Straight after a meal.
- If you are using essential oils, do not have a massage after a hot bath, steam bath or sauna. The body will be eliminating toxins and will not absorb the benefits of the oils.
- Avoid massage on areas where there are bruises, fractures, broken skin, sprains, swellings, rashes, varicose veins, torn muscles or ligaments.

Aromatherapy: The sweet smell of de-stressing

Aromatherapy harnesses the healing power of plant essences. Essential oils are produced from tiny glands in the petals, leaves, stems, bark and wood of many plants and trees. The first recorded therapeutic use of plant oils in Britain was in the thirteenth century, but they also appear in the earliest Chinese records. However, it was a French professor, René Gattefosse, an inventor of perfumes, who revived an interest in essential oils in the early twentieth century. He accidentally plunged his badly burned hand into some lavender essence, instead of water, to cool the pain and found the burn healed without leaving a scar. He then went on to discover many other healing oils.

Essential oils are used by aromatherapists in a variety of ways. In addition to their use in massage, they can be inhaled, added to baths or used in compresses. They are either absorbed through the skin pores and hair follicles, or through the body's olfactory system – that is, via the nose. When the cells in the nose capture odour molecules, signals are sent to the brain's limbic region – the part that governs emotions, behaviour and memory. This area of the brain also ensures our survival and controls the automatic and vital functions of our body, such as adjusting and maintaining the body's heart rate, blood pressure and breathing. When the five senses send messages through the spinal cord it is the reticular activating system (RAS) that filters these stimuli and decides what reaction is required. For example, if you smell smoke, the RAS may raise your heartbeat and send a message to your brain warning you to think about the risk of fire. If you smell lavender, your brain sends signals to your body, via the RAS, to relax. By understanding how the function of smell and touch work in the body, we can see how essential oils and their healing scents and qualities can offer a most fragrant form of relief to even the most stressed-out person!

Are oils safe?

Aromatherapy is thought to be safe and suitable for home use provided you follow the instructions on the bottle. (Refer to Appendix 2) However, any concentrated oils must be used with care as they can cause allergies or skin damage. Here are some guidelines:

- Only buy high quality oils from a specialist aromatherapy supplier. The contents must be pure and this should be stated on the label. Sometimes they are diluted with vegetable oil or alcohol, which affects their potency, but this will be stated on the label.
- Never apply essential oils directly to the skin; they should be mixed with a carrier oil.
- Never swallow any oils unless supervised by a qualified aromatherapist. To find a qualified therapist contact the International Federation of Aromatherapists, 4 Eastmearn Road, West Dulwich, London SE21 8HA, **www.ifaroma.org/**
- Do not be afraid to mix oils; sometimes they work better when more than one is used.
- If you are pregnant, do not use juniper or cedar wood oils, and check with a qualified aromatherapist as to which oils are suitable.

Different ways of using essential oils:

Baths: Adding essential oils to a bath can be extremely therapeutic and work well for muscular aches and pains, tension, fatigue and insomnia. Add 5 to 10 drops of your chosen oil, mix well around the bath - then lie back and enjoy.

Burning oils: Add a few drops of oil to a dish of water set on a radiator or placed in the sun and let the heat evaporate the vapours into the room. Alternatively, invest in an essential oil burner that uses a tea light to heat the water and oil. Remember never to leave a candle in a room unattended, in case of fire. Oils can be used to relax your senses or, in the case of oils such as eucalyptus or pine, to freshen a room.

Inhalants: Excellent for relieving tension headaches, colds and sinus problems. The aroma goes straight to the brain and the therapeutic qualities of the oils to the lungs and then into the blood stream. Put 5 to 10 drops of oil in a bowl containing 570ml of hot water. With a towel covering your head inhale the steam for 5 to 10 minutes. Repeat once or twice a day. Do not try this, if however, you are an asthmatic!

On pillows or handkerchiefs: Put 5 to 8 drops on your pillow at night or on a handkerchief that you can sniff throughout the day. Lavender, in particular, helps you to sleep!

Potpourri: Add your favourite essential oil to top up your fading potpourri and keep the smell alive for longer.

Saunas: Add 2 drops of pine or eucalyptus oil to the ladle of water that is added in saunas to create more steam. This is very pleasant and has antiseptic qualities.

Lavender heating pads: heating pads that are filled with lavender and popped into the microwave for warming are a soothing way to relieve tense muscles. Add a couple of drops of lavender before heating up and the smell will help the relaxing process.

Yoga: Yoking mind and body

The word yoga is Sanskrit for 'yoke' or 'union' and is a technique for combining – or yoking – the spiritual, mental and the physical aspects of life. Practised in India for 4,000 years, yoga was once restricted to a small elite who lived and meditated apart from the world, passing on their knowledge to a few devoted followers. Today it has millions of practitioners all around the world.

Many people in the West concentrate on the postures and exercises called Hatha Yoga, but originally yoga was divided into eight parts. Parts one and two concentrate on conduct, whilst parts three and four form the physical exercises that aim to calm and energise the body and mind. The remaining four parts concentrate on developing mental and spiritual qualities. Hatha Yoga is the most common technique, but there are many variations.[8]

Yoga can be extremely beneficial for those suffering from tension or stress as it is an effective way of stretching and relaxing tensed muscles. Researchers at the Richard Stockton College in New Jersey found that yoga benefited participants with chronic lower back pain, a common complaint often associated with stress.[9] Half of the 22 participants received immediate yoga intervention and the results showed that yoga helped improve balance and flexibility and decreased disability and depression in the yoga intervention group. The Yoga Biomedical Trust, after conducting a poll of 2,000 people, discovered that yogic exercise was extremely beneficial for a number of conditions related to stress: 94% of those suffering from anxiety found that yoga helped them, while the results for insomnia (82%) and high blood pressure (84%) were almost as encouraging. (See Appendix 3)

Yoga can also be used as an excellent way of preventing stress: studies have shown that it is beneficial for over-all physical fitness – the fitter and more supple the body, the less tense the muscles. Researchers at the Department of Exercise Science at the University of California found that regular Hatha Yoga improved muscular strength and endurance, flexibility, cardio-respiratory fitness, body composition and pulmonary function.[10] Researchers in India also found that the practice of Hatha Yogic exercises helped to improve aerobic capacity.[11]

More research is needed, but studies so far have indicated that yoga can benefit sufferers of depression. One recent study of 12 caregivers who looked after patients with dementia showed significant reductions in depression and anxiety, plus improvements in perceived self-efficacy following six sessions of yoga meditation.[12] In another study, 28 volunteers aged 18-29, who were suffering from mild depression with no previous diagnosis or treatment, participated in a yoga course. The results showed participants had significant decreases in their symptoms of depression as well as lower levels of fatigue and fewer negative moods.[13]

The Yoga Biomedical Trust poll of 2,700 people who practised yoga found that over 70% said yoga improved everything from ulcers to haemorrhoids.[14] And we have yoga to thank for the talents of one person in particular. Sir Yehudi Menuhin, the famous violinist, found that practising yoga exercises cured the frozen shoulder that once threatened his brilliant career!

Techniques:

Hatha Yoga: This is one of the most popular traditions in the West, as many followers concentrate only on the postures. Hatha Yoga consists of physical exercises that challenge and refine flexibility, strength and balance. Controlling breathing is an important part of yoga, and this is achieved while focussing on particular postures.

Iyengar Hatha Yoga: This uses props such as blocks, chairs, blankets and belts to help participants reach certain postures safely. Iyengar Hatha Yoga is meditation in action. Students learn postures while focusing the mind on the breath.

As mind unites with body, meditation naturally follows and the whole body relaxes.

Pilates: A new twist to yoga

Pilates (pronounced pil-aah-teez) was invented by a German named Joseph Pilates in the early twentieth century and is a modern variation of yoga. Pilates selected the most effective aspects of yoga, gymnastics, skiing, self-defence, dance and even circus training to work out an exercise system that gave the body a perfect balance of strength and flexibility. He devised many of his forty-plus mat programmes while he was interned in England during the First World War.

Today, Pilates exercise continues to evolve and is less about *what* you do and more about *how* you do it. Pilates himself never set up an official, one-size-fits-all training programme, instead devising unique programmes for individuals. Like yoga, Pilates stretches and exercises tense muscles and is seen as an effective tool in the management of stress. To find a qualified instructor refer to The Body Control Pilates Association, **www.bodycontrol.co.uk.**

Yoga and Pilates Tips:

- Take lessons from a qualified yoga or Pilates instructor.
- If you are taking medication or have a disability or physical condition, consult your doctor before taking up yoga.
- Do not practise yoga or Pilates after a heavy meal. Wait three hours after a meal and one hour after a snack.
- Do not practise yoga or Pilates with a full bladder or bowels.
- Do not compete with others as yoga or Pilates should be individualistic to suit your needs. Yoga and Pilates are not competitive sports!
- Practise regularly but stop if you have a pain or find the moves uncomfortable.

Meditation: It's all in the mind

Meditation has been practised for thousands of years throughout India and Asia as a way of achieving spiritual enlightenment. However, in recent years it has become popular in the West as a self-help method of using your own powers of concentration to control thoughts in order to calm the mind and slow the body – a technique so important with today's busy, frenetic lifestyles.

Over 1,000 studies have been conducted proving that meditation can benefit physiological and psychological health. One such study, conducted at the University of West Virginia, found that out of the 103 adults who completed an 8-week group stress reduction programme that included meditation, 24% reported a decrease in daily stress, 44% reported a decrease in psychological distress and 46% reported a decrease in medical symptoms. These results were maintained when tested again three months later.[15]

Meditation has also been found to reduce blood pressure. Researchers at the Medical College of Georgia taught transcendental meditation (TM) to 50 African-American adolescents with high blood pressure and asked them to practice it for 4 months. Compared to the control group who did not participate in meditation, the TM group showed a significant decrease in blood pressure.[16]

Another study among patients with HIV who participated in a structured 8-week mindfulness-based stress reduction programme that included meditation techniques, found that the activity and numbers of their natural killer cells increased significantly. The researchers concluded that meditation can help strengthen the immune system, but recognised that more research was needed.[17] Meditation has also been found to help people suffering from stress. Canadian researchers studying breast and prostate cancer patients discovered that meditation not only enhanced quality of life, but also showed a decrease in stress symptoms resulting in beneficial changes in hypothalamic-pituitary-adrenal (HPA) axis functioning.[18] Another study that looked at post-traumatic stress disorder in post-war Kosovan high school students showed significant decreases in stress symptoms in all of the 139 students who participated in a 6-week programme that included meditation.[19]

These studies merely skim the surface of masses of evidence pointing towards meditation being a useful tool in managing stress and maintaining health. To summarize the findings, research has shown that meditation:

- lowers oxygen consumption
- decreases respiratory rate
- increases blood flow
- slows the heart rate
- leads to a deep level of relaxation
- decreases blood pressure in people who have normal or mildly elevated pressure
- lowers levels of blood lactate (which is associated with anxiety)

Techniques of meditation

Transcendental Meditation: There are many different techniques and styles of meditation, but Transcendental Meditation is probably one of the best-known since the Beatles and other pop stars became followers in the 1960s. The aim of TM is to quiet the mind so it reaches a 'restful alertness'. By sitting on a chair with your eyes closed, your attention is focused inwards and you learn to think of nothing. There is no chanting, hypnotism, concentrating on a candle flame or religious icon, as in some other techniques, and this simplicity may explain its popularity. Once the technique is learnt, TM can be practised anywhere, from a group meditation in a peaceful room to the carriage of a crowded train. For more details, see the web site **www.t-m.org.uk.**

Here are some further meditation techniques you can try.

Breathing: Focus on your breath as you meditate. Inhale deeply 3 or 4 times, hold your breath for 5 seconds, then exhale deeply. Whenever your concentration wanders, gently return to the rhythm of inhaling and exhaling. Gradually you will feel a change throughout your body and you will become less aware of your breathing, more 'centred' and less captured by your thoughts.

Mantra: It is believed that sounds have vibrations that can be conducive to meditation. Close your eyes and focus on a word or phase that has meaning to you. Repeat this word in your mind with each exhalation. If your mind wanders, return it to the word.

Visualizing a safe place: With closed eyes and steady breathing, visualize yourself in a beautiful place surrounded by nature. It can be a forest, a beach or a beautiful meadow, but must be somewhere that has meaning to you. Smell the fragrances and listen to the sounds of the birds. Watch the clouds dance. Feel that you are part of this beauty and know that you can meditate in this place at any time you want.

Listening: Close your eyes and breathe deeply. As your mind quietens, listen to the sounds around you. Listen with your ears and with your heart. Focus on these sounds and gradually you will not hear anything as you flow towards your centre of being. You can play soothing music while you meditate in this way.

Connecting: With your eyes closed and breathing regulated, visualize clean white light pouring from above into the top of your head and throughout your body, cleansing every cell. Imagine each cell is alive and bright with this powerful light.

Tips:

- There is more that one way to meditate, so experiment to find what suits you. Do not be afraid to mix techniques.
- Join a meditation group – it's often easier when someone talks you through it.
- Do not eat or drink for up to thirty minutes before meditating.
- Choose a quiet room where you will not be interrupted.
- Sit upright in a comfortable chair or on the floor if you prefer.

- If unwanted thoughts come during meditation, merely acknowledge them and resume concentration on your chosen focus.
- Maintain a state of meditation for at least 10 minutes.
- Drink a glass of water straight after meditating as helps you become alert.

Exercise: A little pain, a lot of gain

The last thing many people feel like doing at the end of a stressful day of work – or before their stressful day even begins – is taking some exercise: a jog, a swim, an hour at the gym. However, exercise relieves tension and stress and makes us feel better. Why? The reason is that endorphins (hormones secreted by the pituitary gland into the bloodstream) stimulate physiological changes. There are different types of endorphin (all of which, taken from the Greek alphabet, sound like American college fraternities or sororities): Alpha, Beta, Gamma and Sigma. Endorphins have an analgesic effect on the body and block pain signals from reaching the brain. They are known as the body's natural painkillers.

Research has shown that the beta-endorphins in the blood have been found to increase as much as five times their resting levels after 30 minutes exercise.[20] Therefore, after moderate exercise the body can experience a flood of wellbeing, even euphoria; this explains why some people become addicted to exercise. But the more intense the exercise, the more the body becomes tolerant to endorphins and the more exercise is needed to feel the euphoria. Moderate exercise can strengthen the immune system,[21] but interestingly, acute exercise can cause the opposite – immunodepression.

Although the cause of depression varies from person to person, research has found that most people with depression have low levels or impaired transmission of the neurotransmitters – serotonin and norepinephrine.[22] Neurotransmitters are chemicals made by the nerve cells in the brain that send messages back and forth between each other. When the normal functioning of these neurotransmitters is upset, headaches, depression and other mental health problems may result. Researchers know that depression is associated with low levels of serotonin, but are not sure whether low levels of serotonin cause depression or whether depression causes low levels of serotonin. They do know that depression can often be lifted by raising serotonin levels, and one way to increase serotonin is through exercise.

These are some of the reasons why exercise can help you cope with the effects of stress; furthermore, the social interaction of some sports and activities may also help you to feel more connected to people and less alone. Finally, exercise temporarily distracts your attention from the cause of your stress and can trigger a sense of achievement outside the work environment. So pick up your tennis racket, reach for your dancing shoes, or get your bicycle out of the shed!

Exercise Tips:

- Walking is one of the safest and most effective forms of exercise!
- If you suffer from heart disorders, diabetes, arthritis, back pain, high blood pressure, dizziness or blackouts, talk to your doctor before beginning a new exercise regime.
- If you feel pain or become breathless, stop and rest.
- Start exercising gently and slowly for no more than 20 minutes to begin with.
- Do not take exercise when tired, ill or feverish.
- Warm up properly to reduce the risk of injury or strained muscles.
- Wait at least two hours after a meal before exercising.

No time to cry?

In her song 'No time to Cry', Iris DeMent movingly laments the death of her father and not having the time to grieve because of the demands of her busy life:

> I've got no time to look back, I've got no time to see
> the pieces of my heart that have been ripped away from me.
> And if the feeling starts to coming, I've learned to stop 'em fast
> cause I don't know, if I let them go, they might not wanna pass
> And there's just so many people trying to get me on the phone
> and there's bills to pay, and songs to play, and a house to make a home
> I guess I'm older now and I've got no time to cry[23]

However, crying is not only good for you but also biologically necessary. 'It is some relief to weep,' wrote Ovid, the Roman poet. 'Grief is satisfied and carried off by tears.' Crying is not just an emotional relief as pent-up feelings are released through the pressure valve of the tear ducts. Crying has positive physical effects too. Over 2000 years ago, the Greek philosopher Aristotle claimed that crying at emotional dramas was a way of 'cleansing the mind'. Scientific evidence now suggests that Aristotle was actually right. Researchers have discovered that crying removes toxic substances from the body much in the same way as perspiration, urine, and the air we exhale.[24] William Frey, a biochemist from the University of Minnesota, discovered the neurotransmitter leucine-enkephalin (an endorphin or natural opiate for pain relief) and prolactin (released from the pituary gland in response to emotional stress) are present in tears. But don't think you can cheat by peeling and cutting an onion: tears from emotional crying have a different chemical content than those caused by an irritant such as onion juice.

So don't be embarrassed if your work-related stress is making you feel like a good cry. Holding in your tears – especially if you are a man – might seem like the brave thing to do, but such 'manliness' is probably more harmful to your body than a bruised ego. It is true that women cry more than men, but according to Dr Frey this is more to do with body chemistry than cultural conditioning. He found that women have much higher serum prolactin levels than men. The hormone prolactin is not only connected to the production of tears but present in breast milk as well. Dr Frey found that until puberty there is no difference in crying patterns between boys and girls. Then, between the ages of 12 and 18, women develop up to 60% higher levels of prolactin than men and consequently cry more.

Having a good cry is a step towards healing a body that is overwhelmed by the 'fight or flight' response to stress. And not only is it is OK to do it, your body actually demands it!

Positive Thinking: Turning your negatives to positives

Rudyard Kipling captured the merits of a positive attitude in the first verse of his famous poem, If:

> If you can keep your head when all about you
> Are losing theirs and blaming it on you,
> If you can trust yourself when all men doubt you.
> But make allowance for their doubting too;
> If you can wait and not be tired by waiting,
> Or being lied about, don't deal in lies,
> Or being hated, don't give way to hating,
> And yet don't look too good, not talk too wise:

If you can do this, Kipling says in the final sentence:

> Yours is the Earth and everything that's in it,
> And – which is more – you'll be a Man, my son![25]

It is not only poets who have been fascinated by the power of positive thinking - sociologists have been too. The American sociologist W.I. Thomas (1863-1947) concluded that 'if men define things as real, they are real in their consequences.' Robert K. Merton (1910-2003) developed this idea further, coining the well-known phrase 'self-fulfilling prophecy'. In other words, if you think you are beaten, you are. If you think negatively, even subconsciously, it is possible that your behaviour will unintentionally be modified so that the negative thought will come true! For example, if you say, 'There is no point in my studying for the exam tomorrow because I'm going to fail anyway', well ... we already know what the result will be, don't we?

Let us look next at how negative thinking can affect your health – how your mind can affect your body. Researchers in Canada found that of 3,500 senior citizens who rated their health poor, more were likely to die during the seven-year study than those who claimed they had excellent health.[26] In another study, 68 women who were about to have a cervical smear were interviewed. Based on the women's attitudes, the researchers attempted to predict, prior to the test, which women were more likely to have cancer. 28 of the 68 women were found to have cancer. The researchers correctly predicted 68% of the cancer patients, based on their hopeless attitude, and 77% of the cancer-free women, because of their hopeful attitude.[27]

Unfortunately, as we have seen in Chapter 2, thinking positively can be an extremely onerous task to someone suffering from work-related stress – someone whose experiences are extremely negative. However, research shows that if you can manage to think positively, resistance to disease can be bolstered and you generally feel better.

Just as positive thinking can play a part in maintaining health, so too can belief and hope. In the mid-1950s, more than 10,000 people requiring a new surgical procedure to provide relief from coronary heart disease were randomly divided into two groups, one being given the correct operation and the other a sham, or placebo, operation. Afterwards, 90% of the placebo patients – who did not know that they had not had the correct operation – reported improvements in symptoms, and 75% thought they were doing better in exercise tests. However, medical evidence told a different story: of those who claimed they felt better, only 20% showed evidence of this, 60% showed no improvement and 20% tested worse than before.[28] Thankfully, nowadays such an experiment on humans would be unethical, but it goes to show that faith can indeed work wonders.

In another study, a faith healer was asked to administer 'absent healing' over a period of time to three patients (one with gall bladder disease, one with inoperable cancer and one with severe pancreatitis), all of whom were unaware of the experiment. The researcher recorded no change in their symptoms. The patients were then told that a highly successful faith healer would be sending healing energy to them at a particular time over several weeks – though this was not true. Interestingly, the gall bladder patient became free of pain for a year; the patient with pancreatitis gained 30 lbs and could leave her bed, which she had previously been unable to do; while the cancer patient was able to return home, her swelling reduced and her appetite increased – and although she died from the incurable cancer 3 months later, her last months were relatively comfortable and active.[29]

Although positive thinking is not infallible, there are many examples of how an optimistic mental attitude can help to cure the body of disease. There are several cases of warts being cured by the mind. Dr Bruno Block, a Zurich physician, kept a 'wart-killing' machine in his office. It was noisy, with flashing lights, and patients were convinced of its ability to cure their warts. Block instructed them to place the affected body part on the machine and keep it there until he said the warts were dead. He then painted the warts with a harmless dye and told his patients not to wash it off or touch the warts until they had disappeared. He had a 31% success rate, which is higher than 'spontaneous regression' and suggests that patient faith once again assists healing.[30] Another study, in Massachusetts, found that 9 out of 17 patients given hypnosis to treat warts discovered their warts either completely disappeared or reduced. This did not happen to the control group.[31]

So how can you use your mind and the power of positive thought to relieve your symptoms of stress? By changing the way you look at the problem, as Sally did. Sally, a physiotherapist, spent months worrying about losing the job she loved because of her bullying manager. She worried whether she would be able to get another job or if she would be given a fair reference. She fretted over personal finances and at the unfairness of the situation in which she found herself. 'After about two months off on sick leave I began thinking, hang on, why on earth can't I get another job,' Sally explains. 'Then I started thinking, do I actually need my manager's reference when I can get others? Then it dawned on me that I was wasting too much energy on the 'what ifs'. Why could I not turn the situation into an opportunity and start the business I had always wanted to do?' If Sally had spent too much time complaining about the unfairness of the situation she could have got stuck in a negative thought pattern. By accepting the situation as it was, she was able to abandon the negative thoughts, find solutions and move on. You too can apply this logic to any situation, whether it is coming to terms with a bullying boss, reducing your workload, or keeping your job.

Tips:

- Accept and acknowledge the cause of your stress. Write it down - i.e., 'I cannot cope with my workload. I keep missing deadlines and this makes me feel anxious, causing me to lose sleep …'
- Believe that there is a solution.
- Have faith you will find it.

And if this doesn't work, ponder on this Swedish proverb:

Fear less, hope more,
Whine less, breathe more;
Talk less, say more
Hate less, love more;
And all good things are yours.

Affirming your worth

Affirmations. What are they and how can they help relieve symptoms of stress? According to the *Concise Oxford Dictionary*, to affirm something is to (i) assert strongly, state as fact; (ii) make a formal declaration. Therefore, to make an affirmation, you either say or write a statement which you sincerely believe to be true.

Affirmations are a way of regaining some control over your life. Stress can affect self-esteem in many ways, causing a feeling of powerlessness – if you let it. Researchers at the College of Nursing at the University of Kentucky used techniques of thought-stopping and affirmations on a group of college women aged 18-24 who were at risk of clinical depression. 92 women were randomly assigned either to using the experimental techniques or to a non-intervention group. The results showed that the women using affirmations experienced a decrease in depressive symptoms and negative thinking and had a greater increase in self-esteem than those in the non-intervention group. This continued for 18 months after the experiment finished.[32]

Remember the definition of the self-fulfilling prophecy. Instead of thinking 'there is no point in studying for my exam because I will fail anyway', how about: 'I have a positive view of the future and am proud to be taking my exams', or 'I will do the very best I can in my exams'.

Ben Zander, conductor of the Boston Philharmonic Orchestra and a teacher at the New England Conservatory in Boston, believes strongly in the power of affirmations and gives each of his students an A grade at the beginning of his course. 'This A is not an expectation to live up to', he tells them, 'but a possibility to live into'.[33] He requests one thing of his students: they must write him a letter post-dated to the end of the course, explaining why they got their A. They must imagine what they gained, the milestones they passed and so forth. They are not allowed to use words such as 'I hope', 'I intend' or 'I will'. Not only do all the students get an A, but using this method they believe they deserve it - and it becomes the reality.[34] They are making positive affirmations and living up to their ideal images of themselves.

Techniques:

Writing it down: Write down a statement outlining what you want to happen in your life. Do this at least 10 times each day. An example is 'I have found a solution to my stress'.

Anywhere and anytime: Whenever an unwanted thought pops into your mind, imagine the image or problem as a dot on a computer screen. Watch the dot as it gets smaller and smaller until it disappears.

Eye candy: Choose a postcard or photograph that means something to you and on the back draw a bubble in the centre. Write a statement of where you see yourself in 6 months or a year's time. Sprouting from the bubble draw lines with more statements about how you imagine life in the future without your present problems. For example:

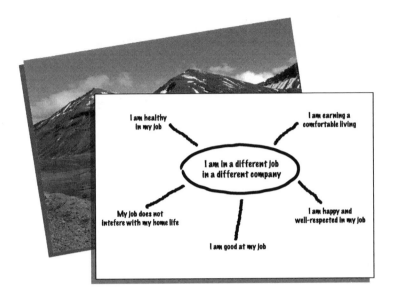

Make several similar cards and place them in visible positions around your house; whenever you pass one, stop and read it.

Exercising affirmations: Repeat your affirmations whilst exercising or taking a walk.

Mirror, mirror on the wall: A technique ideal for those whose self-esteem has been battered. Stand in front of the mirror and make a positive statement about yourself, such as: 'I am a valuable and important person worthy of respect', or 'I have pride in everything I do'.

Bin it: Write down any situations or conversations that have upset you, then tear them up and throw them in the bin. This is excellent for getting rid of negative thoughts.

Affirmations should be personal and relevant to you, but here are some examples to get you started:

- I take charge of my life
- I am healthy
- I am happy
- I am respected
- I am a success in whatever I do
- I treat everyone with consideration and respect
- Negative words cannot hurt me

Re-discover your 'joie de vivre'

According to Dr Olga Gregson from Manchester Metropolitan University, looking at a beautiful painting can actually reduce stress levels and even raise your mood! That is why in 2004 the Manchester City Art Gallery introduced the 'tranquillity tour' aimed at city-centre office workers, allowing people to spend their lunch hour 'chilling out' by looking at hand-picked paintings.[35] The tour takes you through several centuries of painting from the early Victorians and pre-Raphaelites to modern abstract art. The paintings on the tour – which include J.M.W. Turner's *Thomson's Aeolian Harp* (1809) and James Durden's elegantly restful, blue and yellow 1920s interior, *Summer in Cumberland* (1925) – were chosen, according to Andrew Loukes, the gallery's curator, because they suggest restfulness. Although art appreciation is personal, some pieces of art appeal to everyone and evoke, through colour and association, particular responses in the viewer.

Visual stimulation has long been known to have beneficial effects on health. Researchers from the University of Delaware studied 46 patients who had undergone gall bladder surgery. Half of them were put in rooms that overlooked trees whilst the others had a view of a brick wall. The patients who looked out onto the trees spent a shorter time recovering in hospital, expressed fewer negative moods and took fewer painkillers than the patients who looked on to the brick wall.[36] So why not visit an art gallery, or take up gardening and grow beautiful plants or flowers - and experience an unexpected stress-buster.

Negative ions: Or why not take a walk? We have already seen in this chapter how exercise can benefit your health and in the process flood your body with endorphins that make you feel happier. And if you can take a walk near a waterfall, up a mountain or on a beach, so much the better! Did you know that the air in these areas is rich in negative ions that have been shown to increase serotonin, the mood enhancing hormone, in the brain? That's why you really *do* feel better in these environments and not just because the poets and painters tell us we should.

Having a laugh: Researchers have estimated that laughing 100 times gives the body a full workout that is equal to 10 minutes on a rowing machine or 15 minutes on an exercise bike.[37] While rocking with mirth, you are exercising your diaphragm, as well as your abdominal, respiratory, facial, leg and back muscles, which can't be bad. Laughter can also bring balance to all the components in the immune system. It reduces levels of the hormones that swing into action when we experience stress, anger or hostility. Stress hormones, as we already know, suppress the immune system, increase the number of blood platelets (which cause obstructions in arteries) and raise blood pressure. Laughing, on the other hand, actually increases the killer cells that destroy tumours and viruses. Gamma-interferon (a disease-fighting protein) also increases, as do T-cells (a major part of the immune response) and B-cells that make the antibodies that destroy disease!

Not only that, have you noticed how laughing often makes you hiccup or cough? In doing so, you are clearing the respiratory tract of mucous build-up. In addition, laughing also increases salivary immunoglobulin A, which fights infections and any organisms entering through the respiratory tract. In other words, laughing is proven to be good for you, so even if you don't feel like it, force yourself to go out of your way and find things that make you laugh: rent a video, visit a comedy club, or simply have a laugh with friends.

Become a pet owner: Fido and Flossie can also relieve your stress and keep it down. Researchers at the Department of Medicine at the State University of New York found that the blood pressure of pet owners was less likely to increase in response to mental stress than that of non-pet owners.[38] Another study looked at patients who were hospitalised with a heart attack or chest pains. The results showed that after one year only 6% of pet owners died compared to 28% of non-pet owners.[39]

Why does study after study show that pet owners live longer than non-pet owners? Perhaps it is because pets give unconditional, non-judgmental love and, importantly, do not give advice. As stress can be caused or exacerbated by our own actions, a non-judgemental stance is comforting. Academics call this 'non-evaluative social support'. Furthermore, in return for their 'non-evaluative support' pets must be fed and watered and, depending on the pet, exercised. This is one more way of moving the focus away from your own problems.

There are so many ways to retrieve your 'joie de vivre'. Take up singing or bell ringing, learn to cook exotic meals and have dinner parties. Start a repetitive hobby such as knitting, crochet or pottery, or just sit outside and gaze at the stars. As Herodotus said: 'If a man insisted always on being serious, and never allowed himself a bit of fun and relaxation, he would go mad or become unstable without knowing it'. Whatever you decide to do, a hobby or interest will help take the focus away from yourself and your problems. Enjoy life, as the saying goes, because there's plenty of time to be dead. Follow this advice and try to get your stress in perspective – see it as a temporary setback, but nothing that can't be rectified, without the help of, among other things, a good laugh or a full-body massage.

8 STRENGTHENING THE BODY

According to the nursery rhyme:

The best six doctors anywhere
And no-one can deny it
Are sunshine, water, rest, and air
Exercise and diet.
These six will gladly you attend
If only you are willing
Your mind they'll ease
Your will they'll mend
And charge you not a shilling.

Although there is certainly some truth in the rhyme, people suffering from work-related stress might need a little extra help to have their minds eased and their wills mended. So far, in the process of de-stressing our weary bodies, we have learnt how to control our anger and ease our insomnia, how to pamper ourselves with an aromatherapy massage and have a good cry. Next our bodies need to be fortified. This chapter is all about strengthening a stressed-out body with nutritious food, vitamins and herbs, supporting the spine (which carries the weight of the world) and boosting the immune system (which fights the bugs), all with the assistance of good sense and some complementary therapies.

Eating nutritiously

An apple a day – or, to be precise, five servings of fruit and veg – really *does* keep the doctor (and the effects of stress) away. The importance of a nutritious diet has been known since at least the 5th century BC, when one of history's most famous doctors, Hippocrates, wrote: 'If we could give every individual the right amount of nourishment and exercise, not too little and not too much, we would have found the safest way to health.'

Before we look at how prolonged stress can interfere with and deplete the nutrients in the body, and how we can fight back with diet and complementary therapies, let us first remind ourselves of the basics. The body needs building materials to keep it functioning properly, and therefore proteins are vital for growth and cell replacement or repair. **Proteins** also play a role in protecting the body against infection. They can be found in:

- meat
- fish/shellfish
- eggs
- nuts
- seeds
- pulses/beans

Carbohydrates provide fuel for energy. The carbohydrates in refined sugar products (cakes, chocolate bars, etc.) release sugar into the bloodstream quickly, giving a rapid burst of energy, followed by a feeling of lethargy; additionally, these carbohydrates can be stored as excess body fat. Complex carbohydrates or starches, on the other hand, take longer to break down, giving a steadier flow of energy. These healthy carbohydrates are found in:

- wholemeal cereals
- wholemeal bread
- wholemeal pasta
- brown rice
- potatoes

The body also needs **fats** to help form the delicate membranes around the cells in the body, and **fibre or roughage** to carry waste products speedily through the digestive system. Fibre can be found in cereals, grains, bran, fruit and vegetables. Furthermore, the body needs tiny amounts of **minerals** – copper, zinc, sodium, calcium and potassium – to carry out essential biochemical activities. **Vitamins** are also necessary to release energy from food in order to sustain blood cells and hormones, and to maintain the health of the nervous system and organs. Finally, **water** is essential to carry nutrients around the body, to lubricate joints, and to dissolve food for digestion and absorption.

So how does stress affect the nutritional needs of the body? When the body undergoes stress it releases hormones such as cortisol, which, among other things, depletes the body of magnesium, a mineral that plays a vital role in the body's use of energy. Cortisol also increases the production of oestrogen, and while the liver can normally deal with a slight rise in oestrogen levels, a poor diet means the liver's ability to do its job of detoxifying and eliminating oestrogen can be impaired. And as we have already seen, too much oestrogen can cause PMS, endometriosis, ovarian cysts, fibroids and menopausal problems. In addition, stress can deplete calcium, which is necessary for healthy and strong bones. In fact, prolonged stress can knock the whole body out of balance, affecting the immune system and laying the individual open to a variety of illnesses and diseases.

In the management of stress, therefore, it is imperative to eat quality food full of the nutrients, vitamins and minerals your body requires for maintaining optimum health. Judith, deputy manager of a nursing home, became addicted to chocolate, coffee and snack food. 'One minute I felt sluggish,' she says, 'and the next completely hyper.' When Judith left her job she joined Weight Watchers to help her lose the two stone she had put on in 12 months. 'They teach you all about food and its benefits, and give you recipes to cook. Not only did I lose weight,' she explains, 'but I felt healthier than I have ever felt.' Food, like love, can stimulate the immune system which needs to work efficiently if it is going to fight the numerous side effects that prolonged stress can cause. So don't skip on meals, or eat too many snacks or drink too much caffeine, when suffering from stress. Instead, give yourself some healthy and nutritious cupboard love.

Fruit, veg – and juice

The government's Eating Healthily campaign of the 1990s means most of us are aware that we need to eat five portions of fruit or vegetable per day. As with proteins and complex carbohydrates, fresh vegetables or fruits contain specific vitamins or minerals that can help to alleviate some of the symptoms of stress. (See Appendix 4.) For example, the B vitamins – in particular B6 – are important for fighting depression, as B6 converts tryptophan (an essential amino acid) into serotonin (the mood enhancer). The only way for the body to get tryptophan is from food as it cannot produce it itself, nor can it be taken as a supplement. Interestingly, in the United States in the 1980s tryptophan was manufactured into a supplement to treat insomnia. However, it was banned in 1990 by the U.S. Food and Drug Administration because eosinophilia-myalgia, a syndrome that causes muscle pain and even death, occurred from contaminated trytophan supplements. Foods that contain the B vitamins (carrots, avocados, bananas, and leafy green vegetables) will certainly help. Tomatoes provide the antidepressant nutrient phenylalanine which can also enhance memory – and memory loss, according to Dr Bruce McEwen, can be triggered by stress.[1] Cabbage, too, contains memory-boosting choline.

Magnesium is a muscle relaxant found in leafy green vegetables and kiwi fruit. Foods containing magnesium can help overcome a panic attack - another symptom of prolonged stress. 99% of calcium should be in the bones and only 1% in the bloodstream (to ensure that the body will react appropriately to a perceived danger). However, too much stress leaches calcium from the bones and, as it cannot stay in the blood, it is disposed on artery walls, joint tissues or in kidney stones. Therefore, foods high in calcium (from oranges as well as leafy green vegetables such as spin-ach and kale) are valuable in order to avoid osteoporosis in later life, especially for someone in a high-pressure job.

Vitamins and stress

Multivitamins: A healthy diet should provide all the vitamins and minerals your body requires. However, modern production methods and pesticides can affect the vitamin and mineral content of the food we eat, so taking a multivitamin tablet daily ensures the body receives the necessary amount.

Vitamin B complex: As we have seen, the B vitamins are important in combating depres-sion and in easing menstrual problems. Researchers have also found that doses of B-complex can reduce the immune-suppressing effects of stress.[2] The B family is water-soluble and is not stored in the body so any excess amounts will be excreted in urine. However, too much B3 can cause low blood pressure, itching, elevated blood glucose, peptic ulcers, and in extreme cases, liver damage. Likewise, high doses of B6 can cause neurological damage. Therefore, never exceed the recommended dos-age on the packet.

Vitamin C: Professor Samuel Campbell of the University of Alabama-Huntsville found that giving rats large doses of vitamin C abolished the secretion of stress hormones,[3] while Dr. Stuart Brody of the University of Trier in Germany found that people in his tests felt less stressed when they were saturated with vitamin C.[4] It has not been proved beyond doubt that vitamin C supplements strengthen the immune system or prevent the common cold; nevertheless, many people believe they reduce the severity of cold symptoms. The most famous exponent of this theory was Dr Linus Pauling, winner of the Nobel Prize for chemistry in 1954. Author of *Vitamin C and the Common Cold* (1970), Dr Pauling took several grams of vitamin C a day – and lived to the ripe old age of 93. He maintained that environmental stress, among other factors, increases our need for micronutrients like vitamin C beyond the recommended daily amount. Too much vitamin C can cause gastric upsets, however, and may put unnecessary pres-sure on the liver, so again do not exceed the recommended daily dosage.

Juicing

One way to ensure your body gets the correct dosage of vitamins and minerals, with all their stress-busting facilities, is by drinking raw vegetable or fruit juices. The ben-efits of juicing are huge:

- Juices nourish the body within ten minutes – whereas vegetables when eaten take longer to move through the digestive tract.
- One glass of juice can count as one of your five portions of fruit and vegetables a day.
- Vegetables and fruit contain carbohydrates essential for energy.
- Vegetables and fruit can protect you from major diseases such as cancer and heart disease. Some have anti-oxidants such as beta carotene, vitamin C, vitamin E and selenium which are nutrients that protect cell membranes from damaging free-radicals.
- Vegetables and fruit have medicinal properties. For example, blueberries contain an effective anti-diarrhoeal agent, whilst ginger is a known cure for motion sickness.

Dr Norman Walker, the man responsible for introducing juicing to Western diets in 1930, cautions that juices should not replace eating fruit and vegetables because of the body's requirement for fibre.[5] However, juicing is a quick way of nourishing the body directly with the vitamins and minerals it needs.

Dr Walker explains that the human body is made up of sixteen elements, such as phosphorus and manganese, and the body becomes imbalanced if it does not contain the correct proportion. If the situation persists, the body can become poisonous and toxaemic. Juices made from fruits and vegetables are the cure for this situation, according to Walker. Ulcers, fatigue, heart trouble, headaches, insomnia and even cancer – all stress linked diseases – can, according to Dr Walker, be alleviated or prevented by drinking fresh carrot juice. Carrots contain vitamins A, B, C, D, E and K and assist in normalizing the entire bodily system. Finally, fresh juices containing vitamin C are vital for maintaining a healthy immune system that can help in the fight against stress. Fruits and vegetables high in vitamin C include blackcurrants, broccoli, cabbage, grapefruit, green peppers, guava, kale, lemons, oranges, papaya, potatoes, spinach, strawberries, tomatoes and watercress.

So why not invest in an electric juicer and experiment with different tastes and combinations of juices? According to Dr Walker, within 15 minutes of drinking them you will start to feel stronger and healthier.

Herbs and supplements

In 1985, the World Health Organisation estimated that 80% of the world population relied on herbs for primary health care.[6] So why is herbal medicine not in the mainstream in the West? Why are we so reliant on man-made drugs rather than pure plants? Firstly, anything put on the market in the West must be tested, at huge cost, for adverse effects. Secondly, there has been very little research into the medicinal properties of plants because a plant itself cannot be patented. To get around this problem, pharmaceutical companies have researched plants for their biological activity and then isolated and patented the active constituent. However, this isolated constituent is often not as powerful as the complete herb.

Economics, therefore, account for one reason why herbal medicine has not been widely accepted by the traditional medical profession. However, you could argue that the division of Western thought over healing methods is embedded in mythology, beginning with Asklepios, the Greek god of medicine who treated the sick with the help of his daughters, Hygeia and Panacea. Hygeia concentrated on healthy living and disease prevention, while Panacea treated the established disease. Followers of Hygeia believed in the power of nature to heal – by using natural herbs – while admirers of Panacea thought their invented written laws (*materia medica*) were the only way to treat an ailing body. Sadly, this division of thought has persisted throughout the history of Western medicine, including the work of the Roman physician Galen in the first century AD. A follower of Panacea, he devised a system of rules and classification based on Hippocratic medicine, that is, on the balance of the four humours – blood, bile, phlegm and choler.

It wasn't until the 1600s that an Englishman named Nicholas Culpeper revived an interest in Hygeia's herbal medicine by recommending inexpensive herbal remedies acquired from the countryside and back gardens. Traditional medicinal treatments such as the use of mercury, bleeding and purging, remained popular, however, on both sides of the Atlantic as late as the eighteenth century despite the fact that they killed more patients than they cured. Blood was thought to carry the impurities of disease and so bloodletting enabled 'bad' blood to be replaced by new, fresh blood. Not everyone, including Molière, the French dramatist, believed in such health practices: 'Nearly all men die of their remedies and not their illnesses,' he wrote, and he may well have been right. The Renaissance painter Raphael died at the age of 37 after his doctors bled him; and more than two hundred and fifty years later the same thing happened to George Washington, who bled to death as his physicians took 80 ounces of blood (about 35% of all the blood in his body) to cure his sore throat!

In the early 1800s, Samuel Thomson introduced a system of herbal medicine, arrogantly insisting that everything anyone need to know could be found in his works. However, instead of gaining a following, his approach, known as 'Thomsonianism', caused a backlash against herbal medicine. By the end of the 19th century, the Electic movement tried to bridge the gap between traditional medicine, Thomsonianism, and herbal medicine, but this attempt ultimately failed. Later, the Rockerfeller Foundation in the United States gave financial backing to traditional medical schools, thus promoting the modern pharmaceutical industry through which vast sums of money could be made.

Fortunately, anyone wishing to use a herbal remedy today does not need to follow the advice of Nicholas Culpeper and cultivate the petals or seeds by observing a 'celestial harmony' and then grinding them with a pestle and mortar. In the UK, there is any number of herbs and supplements that can either be bought over the counter in health food shops or from qualified herbalists. The recommended dosage will be on the labels. However, if you have any concerns, talk to your doctor.

Alternatively, you could make an appointment to see a Western Herbalist, a practitioner of Traditional Chinese Medicine, or an Ayurveda practitioner. All three healing traditions administer herbs and most practitioners are well trained and experienced in their field. Presently, there are no standard qualifications or training in these healing methods but directives from Europe are working towards statutory registration for Western, Chinese and Ayurvedic herbal traditions. In the meantime, always check qualifications; most will belong to a professional body such as the National Institute of Medical Herbalists (NIMH)[7] or will have trained at a well-known establishment abroad. Below is a brief outline of the different traditions of herbal healing; all can offer remedies for stress and its symptoms:

- *Western Herbalism/Phytotherapy:* This is a holistic approach to healing using plant medicines to relieve illness and promote health. To qualify as a member of the National Institute of Medical Herbalists (uk) (NIMH) herbalists must complete an accredited course and 500 hours of clinical training. To find a registered practitioner refer to the web site **www.nimh.org.uk**.

- *Traditional Chinese Medicine:* Based on the concepts of yin and yang, this type of treatment aims to restore the fundamental balance and harmony between the two. The causes of disease are categorized into three concepts: (i) external diseases caused by bacteria, viruses and unusual weather changes invading the surface of the body; (ii) internal diseases caused by emotional distress, constitutional weakness, toxins, physical stress and exhaustion; and (iii) non-external and non-internal diseases due to improper food intake, irregular diet, traumatic injuries and insect bites. There are more than 3,000 registered products that Chinese herbalists use. To find a registered practitioner refer to the web site **www.rchm.co.uk**.

- *Ayurvedic herbal tradition:* Evolving in India between 3000 and 5000 years ago, Ayurveda is a holistic system of healing that aims to promote harmony between the individual and nature. It focuses on establishing and maintaining the balance of 'life energies' rather than dealing with individual symptoms. It recognises that everyone has a unique constitution requiring different healing regimes. For sufferers of stress, an individual programme of diet, exercise and lifestyle changes are offered. For more information about Ayurvedic medicine refer to the web site **http://niam.com/corpweb/defintion.html** and to find a registered practitioner **www.rchm.co.uk**

Listed below are some of the common oral herbs, vitamins and supplements that are presently available over the counter to treat symptoms of stress and depression. If you are already taking an antidepressant or any other medication, always talk to your doctor first before taking supplements. In some instances, the two do not mix and can cause adverse reactions.

Herbs:

Panax Ginseng (Korean or Chinese ginseng)
For Stress and Fatigue: Ginseng enhances the ability to cope with stress and delays the alarm phase in the 'fight or flight' response. It works on the adrenal glands, which secrete hormones during stress.[8]

Siberian Ginseng
For Stress and Fatigue: Since 2000 BC the Chinese have been using Siberian ginseng which although of the same plant family, differs from Panax ginseng. Researchers concluded, after administering Siberian ginseng to 2,100 people that they could cope better with adverse conditions such as heat, noise, motion, workload increase and exercise. They also showed signs of higher mental alertness and the quality of their work improved.[9]

Valerian
For Stress, Anxiety and Insomnia: A herb with pinkish flowers often seen growing in the wild, valerian acts as a sedative in states of agitation (anxiety) and also, conversely, as a stimulant in extreme cases of fatigue. One study showed that valerian significantly reduced insomnia and improved sleep quality but also had none of the after effects – such as the morning-after grogginess – of barbiturates or benzodiazepines.[10]

St John's Wort
For Depression and Sleep Disorders: This herb, with its yellow flowers, grows all over Europe and the United States, and some people prefer it to traditional antidepressants for treating mild depression. Countless studies have proved that St John's Wort is as effective in relieving symptoms of depression as traditional antidepressants.[11]

Ginko Biloba
For depression: Ginko biloba is a deciduous tree that can live up to 1,000 years. It is traded in Europe under the names of Tanakan, Rōkan, Ginkgobil, Kaveri and Tebonin, and it is the leaves that are used for medicinal purposes. Studies have shown ginko biloba to have antidepressant effects,[12] and forty-four studies involving 9,772 patients showed toxic reaction to ginko biloba to be extremely rare.[13]

Echinacea

For enhancing the immune system: The pink-petalled echinacea grows in Europe and North America, and all nine species of the plant have medicinal properties. Echinacea can positively stimulate different aspects of the immune system, whose function is to protect the body against infection.[14] Sufferers from stress often get frequent colds, and recent studies offer considerable support for using Echinacea as a remedy.[15]

Supplements:

Omega 3 oils: Found in mackerel, salmon, sardines and some plants such as avocados and rapeseed, Omega 3 oils are essential fatty acids and are required for the healthy functioning of the body. However, Western diets contain very few Omega 3 fatty acids, as hydrogenation – the process giving foods a long shelf life – removes them. If Omega 3 oils are low, researchers have found evidence of depression and even bipolar disorder.[16] A recent study in Durham found that 40 out of 100 children showed improved concentration and learning ability after taking Omega 3 capsules for six months;[17] another study found the oils effective in blunting the stress response.[18] Sufferers from stress often experience concentration and memory problems in addition to depression, so taking Omega 3 supplements may be beneficial.

Chiropractic

According to the Health and Safety Executive (HSE), musculoskeletal disorders (MSDs) are the most common occupational illness in the UK, with 1.1 million people affected every year.[19] Many of these have exclusively physical causes, but studies have shown a clear link between work-related stress and musculoskeletal problems. Researchers at the University of Manchester interviewed 896 subjects, all in their twenties and new to the job market, to find out if there was a correlation between musculoskeletal pain and taxing labour and/or lack of job satisfaction. The study examined 12 different work environments and jobs ranging from the physically demanding and dangerous to the comparatively safe, albeit not without pressure and stress. The researchers found that the most significant physical risks were pulling heavy weights and prolonged squatting, but they also discovered a strong link between widespread pain and two psychosocial factors related to stress: low social support and monotonous work.[20]

The HSE also supports the view that stress at work and back pain can be related, stating that psychosocial factors such as high workloads, tight deadlines and lack of control of the work and working methods can lead to musculoskeletal problems. Psychosocial risk factors, such as those mentioned in the Manchester study, may affect workers' psychological response to their work and workplace conditions, thereby leading to increased muscle tension. And tight muscles can, the HSE warns, make someone more susceptible to musculoskeletal problems.

This is exactly what happened to Steve, the researcher in a London borough council. After becoming totally disillusioned with his job, feeling bored and unappreciated, he experienced severe neck and back pains for the first time in his life. 'My doctor couldn't find anything wrong with me, so recommended a local chiropractor. Not knowing what to expect, I made an appointment,' he explains. 'It was slow but remarkable progress. Apparently, slumping over the computer all day without taking breaks did not help my neck, which was already tense, so in addition to the adjustments that were made, my chiropractor gave me stretching exercises to do whilst at work.'

Steve's progress is typical of the experience of many chiropractic patients. A study published in the *British Medical Journal* in 1990 showed just how effective chiropractic treatment can be.[21] 741 patients aged 18-65 were allocated to either chiropractic treatment or hospital outpatient care for their lower-back pain. Outpatient treatment consisted of physical therapy, corset wearing and exercises. The results showed that chiropractic patients enjoyed more long-term benefits for up to two years after treatment. In 1995, the *British Medical Journal* published a follow-up study that showed chiropractic patients reporting less pain than the hospital out-patients and 29% greater over-all improvement.[22]

Spinal manipulation was first recorded in China around 2700 BC, and Hippocrates and Galen, the ancient physicians, were reputed to have practised it. Indeed, Hippocrates even invented a traction machine for stretching the spine! However, spinal manipulation as we know it today is a fairly new medicinal practice dating back to 1895, when a 'magnetic healer' named Daniel David Palmer restored a man's hearing by adjusting some small bones in his back that had become misaligned. The man in question told Palmer that 17 years previously he had felt something move in his back, followed by pain and loss of hearing. On examining the man, Palmer found a painful vertebra in his upper spine. The doctor thrust it back into place and the man, to his amazement, regained his hearing. The Palmer School of Chiropractic – from the Greek *kheir*, meaning hand, and *pratikos*, meaning practical – was founded soon after. Chiropractors today follow in the Palmer tradition, skilfully using their hands to correct disorders of the joints, muscles and spine.

Chiropractors believe that accumulated stresses from emotional as well as chemical and physical sources result in subluxations – minor misalignments in the spinal column that cause nerve interference in the neuro-musculoskeletal system. This reduced nerve flow can adversely affect posture, muscle tone, circulation, the perception of pain, and systemic recovery from stress. By correcting any spinal misalignments, chiropractors can remove accumulated stress from the spine and nervous system, allowing healing to commence. McTimoney chiropractic, using slightly different techniques, is also becoming popular. John McTimoney trained to be a chiropractor in the late 1940s and over the years developed his own technique. Using some of Palmer's methods, the McTimoney technique is gentler, allowing the patient's body to assist in the healing without forcing or stressing the joints or the body.

It is entirely a personal preference as to which technique is more suitable. All chiropractors operating in the UK, including McTimoney practitioners, must be registered with the General Chiropractic Council (GCC) and will have taken an approved course of study. Training takes three to four years, followed by one year supervised clinical practice. To find a registered chiropractor in your area, refer to the web site **www.chiropractic-uk.co.uk/**. For a McTimoney chiropractor refer to **www.mctimoney-chiropractic.org.**

Acupuncture

Acupuncture has been practised in China for over 3,500 years, but it is still viewed with some scepticism in the West despite, for example, television footage of patients undergoing surgery with no anaesthetic other than acupuncture. However, the World Health Organisation (WHO) states that, according to hundreds of clinical trials, there are 28 known health conditions that can be successfully treated with acupuncture.[23] Six of these conditions are often associated with symptoms of stress. They are:[24]

- Depression (7 clinical trials)
- Dysmenorrhoea (menstruation pain) (3 clinical trials)
- Digestive disorders, such as peptic ulcer, chronic gastritis, gastro-spasm, nausea and vomiting (14 clinical trials)
- Headache (10 clinical trials)
- Cardiovascular disorders such as hypertension, hypotension and stroke (9 clinical trials)
- Locomotive disorders such as sciatica, low back pain and neck pain (24 clinical studies)

Acupuncture is based on traditional Chinese medicine. Acupuncturists maintain that an imbalance between the opposing yet complementary forces of yin and yang can cause disease. Treatment is based on the principle that the body's energy, or Qi (pronounced Chee), can become blocked, and that blockages can be treated by sticking needles into the skin at particular points along the meridians - energy channels that run throughout the body, linking the internal organs. Needles are often used with 'moxibustion', the burning of selected herbs (moxa) on or over the skin. Or sometimes 'cupping' is administered, whereby special cups are placed on the skin and warmed to stimulate the acupuncture point.

When the body is stressed, acupuncturists believe, it becomes tense, causing the

Qi to get stuck. As this stuck Qi builds up, it looks for an escape valve, often causing tension headaches and high blood pressure. Stressed people can also get stomach or irritable bowel syndrome when the Qi cannot move through the intestines. Acupuncture helps to smooth the flow of blocked Qi wherever it has built up in the body.

Acupuncture is also known to decrease the stress hormone cortisol, lower blood pressure, reduce the heart rate and relax muscle tissue, as well as to release endorphins – the body's own natural painkillers – whilst improving the circulation of the blood and lymphatic fluids, and thereby bringing fresh oxygen to body tissues.

What to expect: On your first visit, which can take up to an hour, a full medical history is taken. If the acupuncturist is not also a qualified doctor, you may be advised to visit one if he or she is concerned about your symptoms. The acupuncturist will look at your tongue and take your pulse (there are 12 different types of pulse) to gauge your state of health.

You will then be asked to lie, fully clothed, on a couch as the acupuncturist inserts needles in the relevant points, leaving them in for 20 – 30 minutes. The needles are extremely thin and lightweight, so much so that patients are often unaware they have been inserted. Occasionally, bruising can occur, but in most cases there are no side effects other than a relaxed feeling as the needles stimulate the release of natural opiates in the body that relieve pain, enhance mood and reduce stress.

Tips:

- Don't wear tight or restrictive clothing when having treatment.
- Do not consume a heavy meal or drink alcohol immediately before or after treatment.
- Avoid vigorous exercise immediately after treatment.

Julia was recommended by a friend to see an acupuncturist for painful periods that she now knows were caused by stress. 'I was more worried about the needles being sterilized properly than how painful it would be. I didn't want to catch AIDs or hepatitis.' However, her mind was soon put at ease as she watched the acupuncturist take out each needle from individually sealed packages and, after use, dispose of them in a container that was collected by a specialist company. Acupuncture did help Julia's painful periods, supporting clinical evidence showing it to be an effective method of management for menstrual pain.[25]

At present there is no statutory requirement for the training and qualification of acupuncturists, but following directives from the EU, the British Acupuncture Council (BAcC)[26] is looking at ways of regulating standards. Check their website for up-dates on this standardisation and where to find an experienced acupuncturist in your area.

Homeopathy

Homeopathy is a therapy that people either believe in wholeheartedly or dismiss as hocus-pocus. Part of the problem lies in the fact that there is no accepted scientific explanation as to why it works. One reader to *The Times* recently wrote, following an editorial in the paper that came out against homeopathy: 'I feel sorry for people who have to wait for science to tell them that something is real before they can believe it ... The "rational" approach to homeopathy boils down to "we can't explain it, therefore it doesn't exist". This is similar arrogance to the "scientific" experts who stoically dismissed the value of fruit reducing scurvy for years. Science eventually caught up and explained what everyone "knew" anyway.'[27]

So what is this therapy called homeopathy that causes such a divide between those that believe and those that don't?

Homeopathy was introduced in 1810 by a German physician, Samuel Hahnemann, and works on the premise that the body knows how to heal itself. Homeopathic remedies are diluted mixtures of water and a substance, which can be a chemical, element, plant or even a poison. Whatever the substance, it is mixed with 99 parts water, then is vigorously shaken. It is then added to another 99 drops of water (a process called "succussing") to produce the remedy, which is intended to stimulate the body's natural healing energy. In homeopathy, paradoxically, it is believed that the more a substance is diluted, the more potent it becomes.

These dilutions are where traditional scientists really get twitchy. The intense watering-down process in homeopathy conflicts with the accepted laws of chemistry, namely Avogadro's Number, which states that any substance becomes untraceable if it is diluted beyond where a single molecule of the chemical can be found. Scientists argue that homeopathic medicines are diluted far beyond Avogadro's Number. Furthermore, pharmaceutical medicines operate under the notion that more is more: the higher the dose, the quicker the cure.

In 1985, the French biologist Dr Jacques Benveniste discovered that water retains a "memory" of things once dissolved in it; yet when his experiments could not be repeated, he lost his reputation, laboratories and funding. However, in the 1990s a consortium of four independent research laboratories in France, Italy, Belgium and Holland, led by Professor Marcel Roberfroid at Belgium's Catholic University of Louvain in Brussels, discovered through their individual tests that diluted water *did* have a memory of the original substance after all.[28]

One explanation of how this 'memory' occurs was discovered accidentally by Shui

Yin Lo, former visiting associate professor in the chemistry department at the California Institute of Technology. He found when performing experiments on improving car engine efficiency that each substance exerts its own unique influence on water. The substance added to water creates a cluster shape and, with dilution and shaking, the clusters grow bigger and stronger, eventually starting to assume a form that mimics the structure of the original substance. When the original chemical can no longer be detected, its image, so to speak, is still there in the water molecules.

According to Dr Peter Fisher, Clinical Director of the Royal London Homeopathic Hospital, there is now 'substantial scientific evidence for homeopathy': a comprehensive analysis published in *The Lancet* in 1997, for example, concluded that its results were 'not compatible with the hypothesis that the clinical effects of homeopathy are completely due to placebo'.[29] Dr Fisher himself concludes that homeopathy 'is difficult to comprehend in terms of science'. Still, something appears to be at work – and there are, after all, more things in heaven and earth than are dreamt of in scientific laboratories.

As with other complementary therapies, homeopathy uses a holistic approach to healing, prescribing treatment on an individual basis. Remedies are prepared on the basis that 'like cures like', and each contains a small amount of the substance that corresponds to the illness. There is no single remedy that cures the symptoms of stress, as the patient's individual circumstances must be taken into account. Many homeopaths will offer a combination of remedies and might ask to see the patient over several months. This approach is preferable to self-diagnosis, though basic remedies that can be bought over the counter include:

- *Nelsons Kali.phos.6c pillules* for mental tiredness from overwork and nervous exhaustion.
- *Nelsons Nat.Mur.30c pillules* for relief of many symptoms brought on by stress.
- *Arnica* for shock and trauma.

Despite traditional scientific resistance to homeopathy, some homeopaths are also medically qualified – doctors and dentists who have taken additional courses – whilst all homeopaths will have undertaken a three or four year course accredited by either the Society of Homeopaths[30] or the Alliance of Registered Homeopaths.[31] To find a qualified homeopath, refer to the web sites of these organisations. Most homeopaths work privately, but there are NHS homeopathic hospitals in London, Bristol, Tunbridge Wells, Liverpool and Glasgow.

Flower remedies

Flower remedies form another 'so-called' therapy that lacks scientific explanation, yet is popular, safe and the remedies are available in high street chemists. The most well known of flower remedies are Bach (pronounced Batch) Flower Remedies discovered by Dr Edward Bach (1880-1936). He developed 38 preparations for numerous disorders, all made from wild flowers and plants. He believed the dew on flowers was 'impregnated' by the sun, giving them medicinal properties.

A medically trained doctor, bacteriologist and homeopath working in London, Dr Bach became increasingly frustrated with orthodox medicine and its focus on curing *symptoms*. He believed the *cause* of the disease must first be addressed, arguing that disease is 'entirely the result of a conflict between our spiritual and mortal selves'.[32] If we are in harmony with our own nature and do the work for which we are individually suited, health and happiness will follow. Disease, his followers believe, is the reaction to interferences, such as the doubt, fear, or indifference implanted in our minds by others.[33]

The remedies were designed to be simple enough for anyone to self-diagnose and use. Dr Bach divided the 38 remedies into seven groups representing the conflicts that prevent us from being 'true to ourselves':

- Fear
- Uncertainty
- Insufficient interest in present circumstances
- Loneliness
- Over-sensitivity to influences and ideas
- Despondency or despair
- Over-concern for the welfare of others

How can Bach Flower Remedies help you when you are suffering from work-related stress? No single remedy can suit everyone, as different personalities and circumstances must be taken into account; however, the remedies are designed to treat the underlying emotions that have caused your individual reaction to stress. They are not harmful and you can combine 6 or 7 of the remedies at the same time if it seems appropriate. If you pick an inappropriate remedy, it will simply have no effect. Furthermore, the remedies will not interfere with any other medication you may be taking!

You can buy Bach Flower Remedies in their undiluted form over the counter in chemists or health food stores. The most popular, known as Rescue Remedy, is already diluted and ready for immediate use in an emergency or stressful situation. Believers claim that Rescue Remedy will help you face a situation in a better frame of mind. Try a couple of drops of Rescue Remedy on the tongue before a difficult meeting – it might just help to calm your anxiety and keep your fears under control, so that the right decisions can be made.

Most chemists that sell Bach Flower Remedies will also have fact sheets or books about each remedy. For more detailed information contact the Dr Edward Bach

Centre in Oxfordshire: Mount Vernon, Sotwell, Wallingford, Oxon, England. Tel: 01491 834678 or visit their web site at **www.bachcentre.com**.

By the time you finish trying out the techniques in this chapter, you will feel better than ever before. 'Our bodies are our gardens,' William Shakespeare wrote in *Othello*, and 'our wills are our gardeners'. So why not make the effort to cultivate your body by incorporating some of these stress-busting techniques into your everyday life? By caring for and nurturing your body like a delicate seedling, it will flourish, enabling you to deal with stress as it arises.

9 CONCLUSION: A SLIP AND NOT A FALL

Pity poor Abraham Lincoln, who knew a thing or two about stress. Before the age of thirty-five he had lost his job as a store clerk in Salem, Illinois, when the business folded; been made bankrupt when his own grocery store, set up with a partner, collapsed and left him with enormous debts; and suffered a nervous breakdown – spending six months in bed – after his fiancée died. Even his career as a politician met with disappointment as he managed to lose eight elections.

Yet Lincoln was nothing if not a persistent man. 'The path was worn and slippery,' he once said of his troubles in life. 'My foot slipped from under me, knocking the other out of the way, but I recovered and said to myself: "It's a slip and not a fall."' Finally, in 1860, at the age of 59, he was elected the sixteenth President of the United States – and became one of the greatest leaders in the country's history.

Workplace stress should be regarded in the same way that Lincoln viewed his numerous calamities: as a slip and not a fall. Work-related stress is a temporary setback and a problem to be solved. It is not a terminal condition. It *is* completely curable.

Another great leader, Sir Winston Churchill, also had many 'slips' in his working life. Despite living to the grand old age of 90, he suffered from ill health, headaches and depression (which he called his 'Black Dog') throughout his life, much of it caused by stress. His wife Clemmie thought he would 'die of grief,'[1] as she put it, when he was forced to resign as the First Lord of the Admiralty after the disastrous Dardanelles campaign in 1915. He also suffered a heart attack brought on by stress whilst visiting President Roosevelt in the White House in December 1941; and by the end of the war he was so exhausted that he had to be carried from Cabinet meetings by marines.[2]

Neither Lincoln nor Churchill was fortunate enough to have access to the many therapies that are available to us today. However, Churchill understood that we need to work to combat stress. Throughout his extraordinary career he painted, built brick walls and wrote numerous books and articles as a way of reducing the effects of stress. He even wrote four volumes on his ancestor the First Duke of Marlborough, who also suffered, as we have seen, from work-related stress. Indeed, Churchill enjoyed these stress-busters so much that in September 1928 he wrote to Stanley Baldwin, the Conservative Prime Minister, reporting that he had spent 'a delightful month – building a cottage and dictating a book: 200 bricks and 2,000 words per day.'[3] This invigorating prescription might not suit everyone – but we all must find our very own stress-buster that we can turn to in trying times.

As we have seen, work-related stress can have harmful effects on our bodies, brains and behaviour. Most insidiously, perhaps, it can change the way we think. Stress can affect the way we view a situation, whether it is our jobs that we regard as tedious and boring or a bullying boss who makes our lives a misery. With all the chemical changes taking place in our stressed-out bodies we can easily slip into a downward spiral, feeling trapped, exhausted and too lethargic to make the necessary changes. It is easy in these circumstances to focus on the awfulness of the situation instead of searching for solutions. However, according to Alexander Graham Bell, the inventor of the telephone, if we are not mindful, we might not see that when one door closes another opens: 'We so often look so long and so regretfully upon the closed door,' he wrote, 'that we do not see the ones which open for us.'

Indeed, every crisis can present us with an opportunity. Why not look at work-related stress in this way? On the one hand you might have a crisis – a problem causing you stress – but on the other hand, this problem could provide an opportunity for you to make some long overdue changes. Not only can you expand your horizons and grow as a person, but you can also explore new techniques like Pilates to strengthen a tense body, or learn to eat the food that helps combat stress. Who would have thought that a good cry eliminates toxins from the body or that a hearty laugh gives you the equivalent of an aerobic workout? Remember that there is always an answer to your problem – an opportunity to be discovered and explored – and if you can't find it on your own, talk to an expert who can help you. Work-related stress does not have to ruin your life. After all, as Benjamin Disraeli said, 'The secret of success in life is for a man to be ready for his opportunity when it comes.' Are you ready for yours?

Appendix 1

THE HOLMES STRESS SCALE

Death of a spouse	100
Divorce	73
Marital separation	65
Jail term	63
Death of a close relative	63
Personal injury or illness	53
Marriage	50
Fired from job	47
Marital reconciliation	45
Retirement	45
Change in health, family	44
Pregnancy	40
Sexual differences	39
Arrival of new family member	39
Change in financial status	38
Death of a close friend	37
Change to a new type of work	36
Argument with spouse	35
Acquiring a mortgage	31
Foreclosure of mortgage	30
Change in responsibility at work	29
Son or daughter leaving home	29
Trouble with in-laws	29
Outstanding personal achievement	28
Wife starting or stopping work	26
Beginning or ending school	26
Revision of personal habits	24
Trouble with boss	23
Change in working hours	20
Change in working conditions	20
Change in school	20
Change in residence	20
Change in recreation	19

Change in social activities	18
Taking a loan	17
Change in sleeping habits	16
Change in eating habits	16
Change in family get-togethers	15
Going on vacation	13
Minor violations of the law	11

Scoring of Life Changes (LC):

Below 150 LC –
  you have a 34% chance of illness or accident within 2 years.

Between 150–300 LC –
  you have a 51% chance of illness or accident within 2 years.

Over 300 LC –
  you have an 80% chance of illness or accident within 2 years.

Source: T.H.Holmes and R.H.Rahe, 'The Social Readjustment Rating Scale', *Journal of Psychomatic Research*, 11 (1967) pp. 213-218

Appendix 2

ESSENTIAL OILS:

NB. If pregnant, do not use any oils without first consulting a doctor or chemist.

Therapeutic uses:	Essential oil
Anxiety	Jasmine, lavender, marjoram, neroli (orange blossom), basil, bergamot, camphor, chamomile, frankincense, geranium, juniper*, melissa, rose, sandalwood
Apathy	Jasmine, rosemary
Backache	Chamomile, geranium
High blood pressure	Clary sage, lavender, lemon, marjoram, melissa
Depression	Camphor, chamomile, jasmine, thyme, basil, bergamot, clary sage, cypress, geranium
Headache	Chamomile, lavender, lemon marjoram, peppermint, rose, rosemary
Insommia	Basil, chamomile, clary sage, juniper*, lavender, marjoram, neroli (orange blossom), rose, sandalwood, ylang ylang
Sedatives	Chamomile, lavender, lemon, marjoram, thyme
Mental fatigue	Rosemary, basil, peppermint
Muscular aches	Eucalyptus, lavender, rosemary, black pepper
Muscle stiffness	Rosemary, thyme
Nerves/panic	Basil, bergamot, cedarwood*, chamomile, geranium, neroli (orange blossom), rose, thyme, juniper*, lavender, marjoram, melissa

* **Do not use during pregnancy.**

Lesley Bremness, *The Complete Book of Herbs. A Practical Guide to Growing and Using Herbs* (London: Dorling Kindersley, 1995)

Appendix 3

**Information from the Yoga Biomedical Trust -
1983 Poll of 2,700 people.**

Disorder	Number of cases	Percentage helped
Back pain	1142	98
Arthritis or rheumatism	589	90
Anxiety	838	94
Migraine	464	80
Insomnia	542	82
Nerve or muscle disease	112	96
Premenstrual tension	848	77
Menopausal disorders	247	83
Other menstrual problems	317	68
Hypertension	150	84
Heart disease	50	94
Asthma or bronchitis	226	88
Duodenal ulcers	40	90
Haemorrhoids	391	88
Obesity	240	74
Diabetes	10	80
Cancer	29	90
Smoking	219	74
Alcoholism	26	100

Patrick Pietroni (ed), *Reader's Digest Family Guide to Alternative Medicine* (London: Reader's Digest Association, 1991), p.375

Appendix 4a

VITAMINS – Sources

Vitamin	Source
A	Liver, fish (cod and halibut), eggs, dairy products, green and orange vegetables.
B1	Wheatgerm, pork and other lean meats, milk, eggs, yeast and dried beans.
B2	Milk, dairy products, eggs, meats, leafy green vegetables, nuts, liver.
B3	Peanuts, poultry, meats, milk, eggs, whole grains, liver.
B6	Bananas, wholegrain bread, meats, eggs, dried beans, nuts, chicken, fish, liver.
B12	Eggs, shellfish, meats, milk, poultry.
C	Citrus fruits, strawberries, blackcurrants, tomatoes, melons, potatoes, sweet peppers.
D	Cod liver oil, oily fish, egg yolk fortified milk and margarines.
E	Vegetable oils, sunflower seeds, nuts, wheatgerm, leafy green vegetables.
K	Leafy green vegetables, soya beans, cereals.
Pantothenic acid	Eggs, dairy products, fish, cereals, pulses, brewer's yeast.
Biotin	Eggs, dairy products, liver, cereals.
Folic Acid	Leafy green vegetables, pulses, liver, yeast.

Health & Healing: The Natural Way (London: The Reader's Digest Association, 1995)

Appendix 4b

MINERALS - Sources

Mineral	Source
Calcium	Dairy products, dried peas, canned sardines and salmon including bones, leafy green vegetables, oranges.
Chromium	Brewer's yeast, wheatgerm, cheese.
Copper	Liver, kidneys, nuts, cocoa.
Fluoride	Fluoridated water, canned fish (with bones).
Iodine	Seafood, eggs, iodised salt.
Iron	Red meat, liver, eggs, dried beans, leafy green vegetables, molasses.
Magnesium	Nuts, bananas, apricots, soya beans,
Manganese	Leafy green vegetables, tea
Potassium	Bananas, meats, potatoes, oranges, dried fruits.
Phosphorus	Dairy products, meats, fish, nuts, whole grains,
Selenium	Seafood, garlic, tomatoes
Sodium	Table salt
Zinc	Oysters, meats, liver, wheatgerm, pumpkin seeds, sunflower seeds.

Health & Healing: The Natural Way (London: The Reader's Digest Association, 1995)

Selected Bibliography

Adams, Andrea, *Bullying at Work: How to Confront and Overcome it* (London: Virago Press, 2000)

Akerstedt, T. et al, 'Sleep disturbances, work stress, and work hours: a cross-sectional study', *Journal of Psychosomatic Research* 53 (September 2002)

Arthur, Sue, *Money, Choice and Control: The Financial Circumstances of Early Retirement* (London: Joseph Rowntree Foundation, 2003)

Berkman, L.F. et al, 'Social networks, host resistance, and mortality: a nine-year follow-up study of Alameda County residents', *American Journal of Epidemiology*, 109 (February 1979)

Blake, Robert, *Disraeli* (New York: St Martin's Press, 1967)

Bremness, Lesley, *The Complete Book of Herbs: A Practical Guide to Growing and Using Herbs* (London: Dorling Kindersley, 1995)

Bunting, Madeline, *Willing Slaves: How the Overwork Culture is Ruling Our Lives* (London: Harper Collins, 2004)

Cox, Tom et al., *Interventions to Control Stress at Work in Hospital Staff* (London: HSE Books, 2002)

Egolf, B. et al., 'Featuring health risks and mortality: the Roseto effect: a 50-year comparison of mortality rates' *American Journal of Public Health*, 82 (August 1992)

Everson, S.A. et al., 'Stress-induced blood pressure reactivity and incident stroke in middle-aged men', *Stroke* 6 (June 2001)

Fauvel, J.P. et al., 'Perceived job stress but not individual cardiovascular reactivity to stress is related to higher blood pressure at work', *Hypertension* 38 (July 2001)

Field, Tim, *Bully in Sight: How to predict, resist, challenge and combat workplace bullying* (Wantage, Oxon: Wessex Press, 1996)

Frankl, Viktor, *Man's Search for Meaning: An Introduction to Logotherapy* (London: Hodder and Stoughton, 1964)

Fuller, Thomas, *Gnomolgia: Adagies and Proverbs. A compilation of proverbs* (London, 1732)

Gao, Duo, *The Encyclopaedia of Chinese Medicine* (London: Sevenoaks Books, 1997)

Gontzas, A.N.V. et al., 'Chronic insomnia is associated with nyctohemeral activation of the hypothalamic pituitary-adrenal axis: clinical implications', *Journal of Clinical Endocrinal Metabolism* 86 (August 2001)

Gordley, L.B et al., 'Menstrual disorders and occupational, stress and racial factors among military personnel', *Journal of Occupational and Environmental Medicine* 42 (September 2000)

Guest, David et al., *Innovative Employment Contracts: A Flexible Friend?* (London: Department of Organizational Psychology, Birbeck College, University of London, 2000)

Hibbert, Christopher, *The Marlboroughs* (London: Penguin Books, 2002)

Hirsch, Donald, *Crossroads after 50: Improving Choices in Work and Retirement* (York: York Publishing Services, 2003)

Holmes, T. and R. Rahe, 'The Social Readjustment Rating Scale', *Journal of Psychomatic Research,* 11 (1967), pp 213-218

Honoré, Carl, *In Praise of Slowness: How a Worldwide Movement is Challenging the Cult of Speed* (New York: Harper Collins, 2004)

Howard, Judy, *The Work of Dr Edward Bach: An Introduction and Guide to the 38 Flower Remedies* (London: Wigmore Publications Ltd, 1995)

Jenkins, Roy, *Churchill* (London: Pan Books, 2002)

Kinchin, David, *Post Traumatic Stress Disorder: The Invisible Injury* (Wantage, Oxon: Wessex Press, 2001)

Kipling, Rudyard, *A Choice of Kipling's Verse made by T.S. Eliot* (London: Faber and Faber, 1962)

Lilliberg, K. et al., 'Stressful life events and risk of breast cancer in 10,808 women: a cohort study', *American Journal of Epidemiology* 157 (March 2003)

Lutz, Tom, *Crying: The Natural and Cultural History of Tears* (New York: W.W. Norton & Company, Inc, 1999)

McClelland, D.C, 'The effect of motivational arousal through films on salivary immunoglobulin A', *Psychology and Health* 2 (1988)

McEwan, Bruce, 'Protective and damaging effects of stress mediators', *New England Journal of Medicine* 338 (1998)

McEwan, Bruce and E. Stellar, 'Stress and the Individual: Mechanisms leading to disease', *Archives of Internal Medicine* 153 (September 1993)

Montagu, Ashley, *Touching: The Human Significance of the Skin* (New York: Harper & Row, 1986)

Murray, Michael T., *The Healing Power of Herbs: The Enlightened Person's Guide to the Wonders of Medicinal Plants* (California: Prima Publishing, 1995)

Neil, Kate and Patrick Holford, *Balancing Hormones Naturally* (London: Piatkus, 1998)

Ornish, Dean, *Love and Survival: How Good Relationships Can Bring You Health and Well-Being* (London: Vermillion, 1998)

Ornstein, Robert and David Sobel, *The Healing Brain: Breakthrough discoveries about how the brain keeps us healthy* (New York: Simon & Schuster, 1987)

Reader's Digest, *Health & Healing the natural way: Eating for Good Health* (London: Reader's Digest Publishing, 1995)

Robinson, Lynne and Howard Napper, *Intelligent Exercise with Pilates & Yoga* (London: Macmillan, 2002)

Smith, Andrew et al., *The Scale of Occupational Stress: The Bristol Stress and Health at Work Study* (London: Health and Safety Executive Publications, 2000)

Smith, Andrew et al., *The Scale of Occupational Stress: A further analysis of the impact of demographic factors and type of job* (**www.hse.gov.uk/research**. 2000)

Stephens, Tina, *Bullying and Sexual Harassment* (Exeter: Institute of Personnel and Development, 1999)

Tackling Work-Related Stress: A Guide for Employees (London: Health and Safety Executive Publications, 2001)

Watson, Roger et al., *Nurses over 50: Options, Decisions and Outcomes* (London: Joseph Rowntree Foundation, 2003)

Williams, Nick, *The Work We Were Born To Do: Find the work you love, love the work you do* (London: Element Books, 2003)

Zander, Rosamund Stone and Ben Zander, *The Art of Possibility* (New York: Penguin Books, 2002)

Useful Contacts

Bullying

- Tim Field's www.successunlimited.co.uk and www.bullyonline.org
- Andrea Adams Trust help-line Tel: 01273 704900 www.thefieldfoundation.org

Careers Advice

- Information, Advice and Guidance www.iag.org.uk
- Graduate careers advisory web site www.prospects.ac.uk

Complimentary Therapies

- Research Council for Complementary Medicine www.rccm.org.uk
- Institute for Complementary Medicine HYwww.icmedicine.co.uk
- The British Register for Alternative Practice (BRAP) www.brap.co.uk
- The Register of Chinese Herbal Medicine (RCHM) www.rchm.co.uk
- British Acupuncture Council (BAaC) www.acupuncture.org.uk
- Foundation for Traditional Chinese Medicine www.ftcm.org.uk
- The Acupuncture Society www.acupuncturesociety.org.uk
- National Institute of Medical Herbalists, UK (NIMH) www.nimh.org.uk
- The British Homeopathic Association www.trusthomeopathy.org
- The Biomedical Trust www.yogatherapy.org
- The Body Control Pilates Association www.bodycontrol.co.uk
- International Federation of Aromatherapists www.ifaroma.org
- Chiropractic www.chiropractic-uk.co.uk
- McTimoney Chiropractic www.mctimoney-chiropractic.org

Counselling and related services

- British Association for Behavioural and Cognitive Psychotherapist www.babcp.org.uk
- British Association of Anger Management www.angermanage.co.uk
- Life-coaching www.coaching-life.co.uk
- British Sleep Foundation www.britishsleepfoundation.org.uk
- Sleep Assessment Advisory Service www.neuronic.com

Discrimination

- The Equal Opportunities Commission Tel: 0845 601 5901 **www.eoc.org. uk**
- The Commission for Racial Equality Tel: 020 7939 0000 **www.cre.gov.uk**
- The Disability Rights Commission Tel: 0845 7622 633 **www.drc-gb.org**
- The Employers' Forum on Disability Tel: 020 7403 3020 **www.employers-forum.co.uk**

Employment Tribunals

- **www.employmenttribunals.gov.uk**
- **www.ets.gov.uk**
- Employment relations section of the Department of Trade and Industry (DTI) **www.dti.gov.uk/er**

Employment issues

- Acas offers free, confidential and impartial advice Tel: 08457 474747 **www. acas.org.uk**
- Trades Union Congress (TUC) **www.tuc.org.uk**
- Health and Safety Executive (HSE) **www.hse.gov.uk**

Managing stress

- **www.howtomanagestress.co.uk**
- **www.teacherstress.co.uk**
- **www.stress.about.com**
- **www.drnorthrup.com**

Reducing expenses

- utility and phone comparisons **www.uswitch.com**
- credit card and loan comparisons **www.unrarelit.com**
- water utilities comparisons **www.buy.co.uk**
- bank comparisons **www.moneysupermarket.com**
- direct debit **www.directdebit.co.uk**
- using less energy in the house **www.ukpower.co.uk**

NOTES

1 WORK-RELATED STRESS: HOW BIG IS THE PROBLEM?

[1] BBC web site News/business/Workplaces Getting More Stressful (14.10.02)

[2] BBC web site News/health/Campaign Aims to Beat Work-Related Stress (17.04.03)

[3] BBC web site News/health/Campaign Aims to Beat Work Stress (17.04.03)

[4] Tom Cox et al., *Interventions to Control Stress at Work in Hospital Staff* (London: HSE Books, 2002), p. 3

[5] BBC web site News/health/Stress: The Effects (25.06.02)

[6] *Tackling Work-Related Stress: A guide for Employees* (London: Health and Safety Executive Publications, 2001), p.1

[7] Christopher Hibbert, *The Marlboroughs* (London: Penguin Books, 2002), p. 271

[8] Robert Blake, Disraeli (New York: St Martin's Press, 1967), pp. 53, 670

[9] Andrew Smith et al., *The Scale of Occupational Stress: A further analysis of the impact of demographic factors and type of job* **www.hse.gov.uk/research/crr_pdf/2000/crr00311.pdf** , 2000), p. 2

[10] **www.bbc.co.uk**/pressoffice '*Now you're talking! Is the NHS coping?*' (24 March 2004)

[11] 'Doctor, heal thyself', *The Times* (21 August 2004)

[12] Andrew Smith et al., *The Scale of Occupational Stress: The Bristol Stress and Health at Work Study,* p.1

[13] Cox et al., *Interventions to Control Stress at Work in Hospital Staff,* p.1

[14] **www.Personneltoday.com**/ (21.10.03)

[15] **www.guardian.co.uk** John Carvel, 'Overtime culture gets worse' (30.09.03)

[16] **www.howtomanagestress.co.uk** Nov 2003

[17] Ibid.

[18] http:ichuddersfield.icnetwork.co.uk (25.11.03)

[19] **www.howtomanagesstress.co.uk** (Nov 2003)

[20] Ibid.

[21] Ibid.

[22] BBC web site NEWS/Health/NHS nurses 'Bullied by Managers' (10.11.03)

[23] See David Kinchin, *Post Traumatic Stress Disorder: The invisible injury* (Wantage, Oxon.: Wessex Press, 2001), pp. 7, 33-5, 42-4

[24] Tim Field, *Bully in Sight* (Wantage, Oxon: Wessex Press, 1996), p. xxiii

[25] Ibid.

[26] BBC Radio 4, *Bullying at Work* (19.12.03)

[27] Ibid.

[28] Nick Williams, *The Work We Are Born To Do* (London: Element, 2002), p. 2

[29] Cox et al., *Interventions to Control Stress at Work in Hospital Staff,* p. 2

[30] Smith et al., *The Scale of Occupational Stress: The Bristol Stress and Health at Work Study,* p.102

[31] David Guest et al., *Innovative Employment Contracts: a Flexible friend?* (London: Department of Organizational Psychology, Birbeck College, University of London, 2000)

[32] Ibid.

[33] *Research on New Forms of Contractual Relationships and the Implications for Occupational safety at Work'* 2002 full report *http://agency.osha.eu.int/publications/reports/206/een/index.htm*

[34] **www.bbc.co.uk/1/hi/business/1530355.stm**

[35] For details of employment legislation, see **www.dti.gov.uk**

[36] **www.statistics.gov.uk/census2001/profiles/cemmentaries/people.asp**

[37] **http://news.bbc.co.uk/1/hi/health/1506209.stm**

2 BODIES, BRAINS AND STRESS

[1] Dean Ornish, *Love and Survival* (London: Vermillion, 2001), p. 24

[2] Ibid, p. 44. In this study, carried out in Sweden, 17,000 men and women between 29 –74 years were followed for 6 years.

[3] D.C. McClelland, 'The effect of motivational arousal through films on salivary immunoglobulin A', *Psychology and Health 2* (1988), pp. 31-32

[4] **www.drnorthrup.com/menopause-11.php**

[5] J. P. Fauvel et al., 'Perceived job stress but not individual cardiovascular reactivity to stress is related to higher blood pressure at work,' *Hypertension* 38 (July 2001), pp. 71-5

[6] S.A. Everson et al., 'Stress-induced blood pressure reactivity and incident stroke in middle-aged men', *Stroke* 6 (June 2001), pp.1263-70

[7] Melissa C.Stoppler, **www.stress.about.com**

[8] L.B. Gordley et al, 'Menstrual disorders and occupational stress, and racial factors among military personnel', *Journal of Occupational and Environmental Medicine* 42 (September 2000), pp. 871-81

[9] BBC web site News/health/stress: The Effects (25.06.01)

[10] K. Lillberg et al, 'Stressful life events and risk of breast cancer in 10,808 women: a cohort study', *American Journal of Epidemiology* 157 (March 2003), pp. 415-23. Over 5,000 sets of twins were questioned in 1975 and then again between 1982-96. Life stresses such as divorce/separation, death of a spouse, close friend or relative were all associated with a significant increase in breast cancer.

[11] Bruce S. McEwen and E. Stellar, 'Stress and the Individual: Mechanisms leading to disease', *Archives of Internal Medicine* 153 (September 1993), pp. 2093-2101; and McEwen, 'Protective and damaging effects of stress mediators', *New England Journal of Medicine* 338 (1998), pp. 171-9

[12] Kinchin, *Post Traumatic Stress Disorder*, pp. 42-4

[13] Robert Ornstein and David Sobel, *The Healing Brain: Breakthrough Discoveries about How the Brain Keeps us Healthy* (New York: Simon and Schuster,1987), p. 247

[14] Arthur Crisp, ed., 'Every Family in the Land: Understanding prejudice and discrimination against people with mental illness' **www.stigma.org/everyfamily**

[15] Symptoms described are from *Diagnostic and Statistical Manual of Mental Disorders*, DSM-IV, 1994

[16] Review Panel on Coronary-Prone Behaviour and Coronary Heart Disease, 'Coronary-prone behaviour and coronary heart disease: a critical review,' *Circulation* (1978), pp. 1199-1215

[17] 'How anger affects your health', *Berkeley Wellness Letter* 8 (January 1992)

[18] **www.apa.org/pubinfo/panic.html**

[19] Smith et al, *The Scale of Occupational Stress: The Bristol Stress and Health at Work Study*, p. 53

[20] T. Akerstedt et al., 'Sleep disturbances, work stress, and work hours: a cross-sectional study', *Journal of Psychosomatic Research* 53 (September 2002), pp. 741-8

[21] 'Sleep-deprived Britain told to catnap its way back to health', *The Sunday Times* (28 December 2003)

[22] A. N. V. Gontzas et al., 'Chronic insomnia is associated with nyctohemeral activation of the hypothalamic pituitary-adrenal axis: clinical implications', *Journal of Clinical Endocrinal Metabolism* 86 (August 2001), pp. 3787-94

[23] "http://www.stress.about.com" **www.stress.about.com**

[24] 'Stress: A Million Claiming Benefits', *Daily Mail* (2 March 2004), p.1

3 WHAT ARE MY RIGHTS?

[1] **www.tuc.org.uk/tuc/rights_joblaw.cfm**

[2] **www.tenant.net/Community/LES/hours10.htm**

[3] BBC web site News/health/Campaign Aims to beat Work-related stress (17.04.03)

[4] National statistics online **www.statistics.gov.uk**

[5] Smith et al., *The Scale of Occupational Stress, The Bristol Stress and Health at Work Study*, p.118

[6] Smith et al., T*he Scale of Occupational Stress*, p.40

[7] **http://164.36.164.20/work-lifebalance/**DTI web site (16.10.03)

[8] Smith et al., *The Scale of Occupational Stress*, pp. 34-5

[9] **www.eoc.org.uk** Tel: 0845 601 5901

[10] **www.cre.gov.uk** Tel: 020 7939 0000

[11] **www.drc-gb.org** Tel: 0845 7622 633

[12] **www.employers-forum.co.uk** Tel: 020 7403 3020

[13] **www.acas.org.uk** Tel: 08457 474747

[14] **www.eoc-law.org.uk**

[15] On your return to work employers will usually give you a standard certificate to fill out asking for the reasons of your absence, and this will then be kept in your personal files.

[16] See **www.dti.gov.uk/er/individual/disres_back.htm**

[17] For details, see **www.acas.org.uk**

[18] **www.businesslink4london.com** Directors' Briefing HR21

[19] Anti-union laws of 1980,1982,1984,1988, 1990.

[20] **www.unionhistory.info**

[21] **www.tuc.org.uk/tuc/rights**

[22] 'Confidentiality: RCN Guidance for Occupational Nurses', (Royal College of Nursing, 2002), **www.rcn.org.uk**

[23] The Terrorism Act 2000, and Anti-Terrorism, Crime and Security Act 2001

[24] IDS Brief, 661, May 2000 **www.idsbrief.co.uk**

[25] Ibid. (Bartholomew v London borough of Hackney 1999 IRLR 246)

[26] Ibid. (Kidd v Axa Equity & Law Assurance Society plc & anor, 2000 IRLR 301)

[27] IDS Brief, 661 May 2000 **www.idsbrief.co.uk**

[28] see **www.kevinboone.com/PF_lawglos_Unfair_Contract_Terms_Act(1977)html**

[29] Thomas Fuller, *Gnomolgia: Adagies and Proverbs. A compilation of proverbs* (London, 1732)

4 TAKING ACTION

[1] Victor Frankl, *Man's Search for Meaning*, trans. Ilse Lasch (London: Hodder & Stoughton,

1964), pp. 65-66

[2] **www.unison.ie/polls**; **http://archives.tcm.ie/breakingnews**; **www.anaova.com/news/story**

[3] **www.news.bbc.co.uk/1/hi/business/229233.stm**

[4] **http://www.tuc.org.uk/law/tuc**

[5] Royal College of Nursing, Confidentiality RCN Guidance for Occupational Nurses, 2002, p. 2 **www.rcn.org.uk**

[6] The Department of Health recommends 8 years, the British Medical Association 10 years (ibid, p. 7)

[7] Royal College of Nursing, 'Confidentiality RCN Guidance for Occupational Nurses,' p. 7

[8] Ibid, p. 5

[9] BBC web site News/health/Campaign aims to beat work stress (17.04.03)

[10] BBC Press office, 'Stressed GPs expect to get more stressed as new contract bites next week' **www.bbc.co.uk/pressoffice** (23.3.04)

[11] B. Egolf et al., 'Featuring health risks and mortality: the Roseto effect: a 50-year comparison of mortality rates,' *American Journal of Public Health* 8 (1992), pp. 889-92

[12] L.F. Berkman et al., 'Social networks, host resistance, and mortality: a nine-year follow-up study of Alameda County residents,' *American Journal of Epidemiology* 2 (1979), pp. 186-204

[13] Dean Ornish, *Love and Survival*, Chapter 2.

5 SHOULD I STAY OR SHOULD I GO?

[1] **www.iag.org.uk**

[2] Quoted in Michael White, *Leonardo: The First Scientist* (London: Little, Brown, 2000), p.108

[3] Web site BBCNews/Education/Debt stress 'fuels student depression'

[4] **http://www.acs.ohio-state.edu/units/research/archive/debthlth.htm** (28.2.00)

[5] Music and words by Dolly Parton, Warner Brothers, 1980

[6] Downshifting –one man's tale (15.10.2003) **http://news.bbc.co.uk/go/pr/fr/-1/hi/wales/3194688.stm**

[7] Donald Hirsch, *Crossroads after 50: Improving Choices in Work and Retirement* (York: York Publishing Services, 2003)

[8] Sue Arthur, *Money, Choice and Control: The Financial Circumstances of Early Retirement* (Joseph Rowntree Foundation, 2003)

[9] Roger Watson et al., *Nurses over 50: Options, Decisions and Outcomes* (Joseph Rowntree Foundation, 2003)

[10] **www.channel4.com/health/microsites/0-9/4health/stress/aas_poll.html**

[11] Richard Morrison, 'A gap year? Don't mind if I do', *The Times* (April 5, 2004)

[12] Op cit.

6 COPING STRATEGIES

[1] Mental Health Foundation, *The Fundamental Facts*, 1999 **www.mind.org.uk**

[2] *The Times* (1 May 2004)

[3] Tracy McVeigh, 'Depression hits one in four adults', **www.society.guardian.co.uk** 8 Jan 2001

[4] Quoted in Hara Estroff Marano, 'Antidepressants: Which drug for whom' (April 2002) **www.psychologytoday.com/htdocs/prod/ptoarticle/pto-20030401-000010,asp**

[5] E.A. Workman et al., 'Atypical antidepressants versus imipramine in the treatment of major

depression: a metaanalysis', *Journal of Clinical Psychiatry* 54 (1993), pp. 5-12; F. Song et al., 'Selective serotonin reuptake inhibitors: metaanalysis of efficacy and acceptability,' *British Medical Journal* 306 (1993), pp. 1124-6; discussion 1126-7

[6] N. Freemantle et al., 'Prescribing selective serotonin reuptake inhibitors as strategy for prevention of suicide', *British Medical Journal* 309 (1994), pp. 249-53

[7] www.cognitivetherapy.com

[8] *Controlling Anger – Before it Controls You*, American Psychological Association www.apa.org/pubinfo/anger.html

[9] William Shakespeare, *Hamlet*, Act 3, Scene 1, lines 1-4

[10] R. Ryan and J. Travis, *The Wellness Workbook* (Toronto: Ten Speed Press, 1993)

[11] Michael Van Straten, *The Good Sleep Guide* (London: Kyle Cathie, 2004)

[12] Ibid.

7 THE 'FEEL GOOD' FACTOR

[1] A. Montagu, *Touching: The Human Significance of the Skin* (New York: Harper & Row, 1986), p. 97

[2] Ibid.

[3] George Anfield ed., *Reader's Digest Family Guide to Alternative Medicine* (London: Reader's Digest Association, 1991), p. 224

[4] www.holistic-online.com/massage/mas_benefits.htm

[5] Ibid.

[6] Ibid.

[7] www.amtamassage.org

[8] For details of these yoga traditions, refer to the web site www.self-realization.com/yoga

[9] M.L. Galantino et al., 'The impact of modified hatha yoga on chronic low back pain: a pilot study', *Alternative Therapy Health Medicine* 10 (Mar-Apr 2004), pp. 56-9

[10] M.D. Tran et al., 'Effects of hatha yoga practice on the health-related aspects of physical fitness', *Preventative Cardiology* 4 (Autumn 2001), pp. 165-170

[11] U.S. Ray et al., 'Aerobic capacity & perceived exertion after practice of hatha yogic exercises', *Indian Journal of Medical Research* (Dec 2001), pp. 215-21

[12] L.C. Waelde et al., 'A pilot study of a yoga and mediation intervention for dementia caregiver stress', *Journal of Clinical Psychology* 60 (June 2004), pp. 677-87

[13] A. Woolery et al., 'A yoga intervention for young adults with elevated symptoms of depression', *Alternative Therapy Health Medicine* 10 (Mar-Apr 2004), pp. 60-3

[14] www.yogatherapy.org

[15] K.A. Williams et al., 'Evaluation of a wellness-based mindfulness stress reduction intervention: a controlled trial', *American Journal of Health Promotion* 15 (Jul-Aug 2001), pp. 422-32

[16] V.A. Barnes et al., 'Impact of transcendental meditation on ambulatory blood pressure in African-American adolescents', *American Journal of Hypertension* 17 (April 2004), pp. 366-9

[17] F.P. Robinson et al., 'Psycho-endocrine-immune response to mindfulness-based stress reduction in individuals infected with the human immunodeficiency virus: a quasiexperimental study', *Journal of Alternative Complementary Medicine* 9 (Oct 2003), pp. 683-94

[18] L.E. Carlson et al., 'Mindfulness-based stress reduction in relation to quality of life, mood, symptoms of stress and levels of cortisol, dehydroepiandrosterone sulfate (DHEAS) and melatonin in breast and prostrate cancer outpatients', *Psychoneuroendocrinology* 29 (May

2004), pp.448-74

[19] J.S. Gordon et al., 'Treatment of posttraumatic stress disorder in post-war Kosovan high school students using mind-body skills groups: a pilot study', *Journal of Trauma Stress* 17 (April 2004), pp. 143-7

[20] 'The antidepressive effects of exercise,' cited 2203 December Neurochemistry **http://sulcus.berkeley.edu/mcb/165_001/papers/manuscripts/_512.html**

[21] D.C. Nieman, 'Exercise effects on systemic immunity', *Immunology and Cell Biology* 5 (2000), pp. 496-501; idem, 'Exercise infection and immunity', *International Journal of Sports Medicine* 15 (1994), pp. 131-141; R.J. Shephard and N. Pang., 'Exercise, immunity and susceptibility to infection', *The Physician and Sports Medicine* 6 (1999), available at **www.physsportsmed.com/issues/1999/06_99/jun99.htm**

[22] J.M. Neal, The Pituitary Gland: *Basic Endocrinology, an integrative approach* (Oxford: Blackwell Science, 2000), pp. 21-22

[23] Iris DeMent, 'No Time to Cry' © 1993 Songs of Iris ASCAP

[24] W.H. Frey et al., 'Effect of stimulus on the chemical composition of human tears', *American Journal of Ophthalmology* 92 (1981), pp. 559-67

[25] Rudyard Kipling, *A Choice of Kipling's Verse made by T.S. Eliot* (London: Faber and Faber, 1963), pp. 273-74

[26] J.M. Mossey and E. Shapiro, 'Self-rated health: A predictor of mortality among the elderly', *American Journal of Public Health* 72 (1982), pp. 800-07

[27] A. Schmale and H. Aker, 'Hopelessness as a predictor of cervical cancer', *Social Science and Medicine* 5 (1971), pp. 95-100

[28] Quoted in Ornstein and Sobel, *The Healing Brain*, pp. 80-81

[29] H. Rheder, 'Wunderheilungen, ein experiment', *Hippokrates* 26 (1955), pp. 577-80

[30] Theodore Barber, 'Changing "unchangeable" bodily processes by (hypnotic) suggestions', *Advances* 1 (1984), pp. 7-36

[31] O.S. Surman et al., 'Hypnosis in the treatment of warts', *Archives of General Psychiatry* 28 (1973), pp. 439-41

[32] A.R. Peden et al., 'Preventing depression in high-risk college women: a report of an 18-month follow-up', *Journal of American College Health* 49 (May 2001), pp. 299-306

[33] Rosamund Stone Zander and Ben Zander, *The Art of Possibility* (New York: Penguin Books, 2002), p. 26

[34] Ibid., pp. 25-53.

[35] 'Forget the gym, there's an art to conquering workplace stress', *The Times* (16 June 2004)

[36] R.S. Ulrick, 'View through a window may influence recovery from surgery', *Science* 224 (1984), pp. 420-21

[37] **http://people.howstuffworks.com/laughter.htm**

[38] K. Allen et al., 'Cardiovascular reactivity and the presence of pets, friends, and spouses: the truth about cats and dogs', *Psychosomatic Medicine* 5 (Sep-Oct 2002), pp. 727-39

[39] E.A. Friedmann et al., 'Animal companions and one-year survival of patients after discharge from a coronary care unit', *Public Health Reports* 95 (1980), pp. 307-12

8 STRENGTHENING THE BODY

[1] Bruce McEwen et al., 'Stress and the Individual: Mechanisms leading to disease', *Archives of Internal Medicine* (September 1993), pp. 2093-2101

[2] N.Y. Ann, *Academy of Science* 58 (1990), pp. 513-5

[3] **http://lpi.oregonstate.edu/f-w99/newresearch.html** (2003)

[4] *Psychopharmacology* 159 (2002), pp. 319-324

[5] Norman Walker, *Fresh Vegetable and Fruit Juices* (United States: Norfolk Press, 1978)

[6] N. Farnsworth et al., 'Medicinal Plants in Therapy', *Bulletin World Health Organisation* 65 (1985), pp. 965-981

[7] **www.nimh.org.uk**

[8] E. Bombardelli, *Chemical, Pharmacological and Clinical Profile* (Milan: Indena S.p.A, 1989); E.V. Avakia and E. Evonuk, 'Effects of panax ginseng extract on tissue glycogen and adrenal cholesterol depletion during prolonged exercise', *Planta Medica* 36 (1979), pp.43-48; and S.J Fulder, 'Ginseng and the hypothalamic –pituitary control of stress', *American Journal of Chinese Medicine* 9 (1981), pp.112-118

[9] N.R. Farnsworth et al., 'Siberian ginseng (*Eleutherococcus senticosus*): Current status as an adaptogen', *Economic and Mediicinal Plant Research* 1 (1985), pp. 156-215

[10] P.D. Leathwood and F. Chauffard, 'Aqueous extract of valerian reduces latency to fall asleep in man', *Planta Medica* 54 (1985), pp. 144-148; H. Dressing et al., 'Insomnia: Are Valerian/Melissa combinations of equal value to benzodiazepine?' *Therapiewoche* 42 (1992), pp. 726-736; and O. Lindahl and L. Londwall, 'Double blind study of a valerian preparation', *Pharmacology Biochemistry and Behaviour* 32 (1989), pp. 1065-1066

[11] P. Morassoni and E. Bombardelli, *Hypericum perforatum* (Milan, Italy: Indena, 1994); U. Schmidt and H. Sommer, 'St John's Wort extract in the ambulatory therapy of depression: Attention and reaction ability are preserved, *Forschr Med* 111 (1993), pp. 339-342; D. Schlich et al., 'Treatment of depressive conditions with hypericum', *Psychology* 13 (1987), pp. 440-444; and G.Harrer and H. Sommer, 'Treatment of mild/moderate depressions with Hypericum', *Phytomed* 1(1994), pp. 3-8

[12] H. Schubert and P. Halama, 'Depressive episode primarily unresponsive to therapy in elderly patients: Efficacy of Ginko Biloba in combination with antidepressants', *Geriatr Forsch* 3 (1993), pp. 45-53

[13] E.W. Funfgeld, ed., *Rokan (Ginko Biloba):Recent Results in Pharmacology and Clinic* (New York: Springer-Verlag, 1988); J. Kleijnen and P. Knipschild, 'Ginko Biloba', The Lancet 340 (1992), pp. 1136-9; J.Kleijnen and P. Knipschild, 'Ginko bilabo for cerebral insufficiency', *British Journal of Clinical Pharmacology* 34 (1992), pp. 352-358

[14] C. Hobbs, *The Echinacea Handbook* (Portland, Oregon: Eclectic Medical Publications, 1989); R. Bauer and H. Wagner, 'Echinacea species as potential immunostimulatory drugs', *Econ Med Plant Res* 5 (1991), pp. 253-321

[15] B. Braunig et al., 'Echinacea purpurea radix for strengthening the immune response in flu-like infections', *Z Phytother* 13 (1992), pp. 7-13; and D. Schoneberger, 'The influence of immune-stimulating effects of pressed juice from Echinacea purpurea on the course and severity of colds: Results of a double-blind study', *Forum Immunology* 8 (1992), pp. 2-12

[16] Four studies have reported a reduced blood level of omega-3 fatty acids in people with depression: M. Maes et al., 'Fatty acid compostition in major depression: decreased omega 3 fractions in cholesteryl esters and increased C20: 4 omega 6/C20: 5 omega 3 ratio in cholesteryl esters and phospholipids', *Journal of Affective Disorders* 38 (1996), pp. 35-46; R. Edwards et al., 'Omega-3 polyunsaturated fatty acid levels in the diet and in red blood cell membranes of depressed patients', *Journal of Affective Disorders* 48 (1998), pp.149-55; M. Peet et al., 'Depletion of omega-3 fatty acid levels in red blood cell membranes of depressive patients', *Biological Psychiatry* 43 (1998), pp. 315-9; and M. Maes et al., 'Lowered omega 3 polyunsaturated fatty acids in serum phospholipids and cholesteryl esters of depressed patients', *Psychiatry Research* 85 (1999), pp. 275-91

[17] **www.bbc.co.uk/science/humanbody/mind/articles/intelligenceandmemory/omega**

[18] J. Delarne et al., 'Fish oils prevents the adrenal activation elicited by mental stress in healthy men', *Diabetes Metabolism* 3 (June 2003), pp. 289-95

[19] www.hse.gov.uk

[20] E.F. Harkness et al., 'Mechanical injury and psychosocial factors in the work place predict the onset of widespread body pain: A two-year prospective study among cohorts of newly employed workers', *Arthritis & Rheumatism* 50 (May 2004), pp. 1665-1664

[21] T.W Meade et al., 'Low Back Pain of Mechanical Origin: Randomised Comparison of Chiropractic and Hospital Outpatient Treatment', *British Medical Journal* 300 (June 1990), pp. 1431-1437

[22] T.W Meade et al., 'Randomised Comparison of Chiropractic and Hospital Outpatient Management for Low Back Pain: Results from Extended Follow-up', *British Medical Journal* 311 (Aug 1995), pp. 349-351

[23] *Acupuncture: Review and Analysis of Reports on Controlled Clinical Trials* (Geneva: WHO, 2002)

[24] Ibid. See references of all the studies on pp. 67-81.

[25] See, for example, J.M. Helms, 'Acupuncture for the management of primary dsymenorrhoea', *Obstetrics and Gyneocology* 69 (1987), pp. 51-56; X.L Shi et al., 'Acupunture at SP6 in the treatment of primary dsymenorrhoea', *Chinese Acupuncture and Moxibustion* 14 (1994), pp. 241-2; and J. Li et al., 'Treatment of 108 cases of premenstrual tension by head acupuncture', *Chinese Acupuncture and Moxibustion* 12 (1992), pp. 245-6

[26] www.acupuncture.org.uk

[27] 'Homeopathy comes under scrutiny', *The Times* (13 September 2004), letter from Richard Stenning.

[28] 'Thanks for the memory', *The Guardian* (15 March 2001)

[29] 'Homeopathy comes under scrutiny', *The Times* (13 September 2004)

[30] www.trusthomeopathy.org/trust/tru_over.html

[31] www.a-r-h.org

[32] J. Howard, *The Work of Dr Edward Bach: An introduction and guide to the 38 flower remedies* (London: Wigmore Publications Ltd, 1995), p. 7

[33] Ibid, p.8

CONCLUSION

[1] 'Working for the common good helped Winston Churchill battle depression', New York City Voices (April/May 2002), found at www.newyorkcityvoices.org/2002aprmay/20020534.html

[2] Roy Jenkins, *Churchill* (London: Pan Macmillan, 2002), p. 788

[3] Ibid, p. 421

ISBN 1-41205465-6

Made in the USA
San Bernardino, CA
14 July 2017